Unlock Your Energy, Confidence, and Joy

Your Menopause Balance

A practical, holistic guide to thriving beyond menopause

By

Luci Harrison

Disclaimer:

The content of this book is intended for informational and educational purposes only and does not substitute professional medical advice, diagnosis, or treatment. The author is not a licensed medical practitioner and does not prescribe the use of any technique as a substitute for medical treatment by a licensed health care provider.

Always consult your doctor or qualified health professional before starting any new health, nutrition, supplement, or exercise program, especially if you have existing medical conditions or are taking medication.

Any application of the information in this book is undertaken at the reader's sole discretion and risk. The author and publisher disclaim any liability for loss or injury resulting from the use of information herein.

This book draws inspiration from real experiences and individuals. However, to protect the privacy of those involved, the names and identifying details of certain individuals have been changed. In some instances, composite characters may have been created from the experiences of several people. Any resemblance to actual persons, living or dead, or actual events is purely coincidental.

Senior Editor: Solveig Dupont

Cover Design: Nada Orlic

ISBN 978-0-473-76648-1

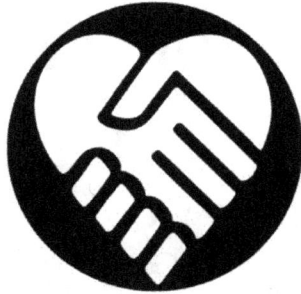

Dedication

To the sisterhood of women rising through midlife together,
this book is for you.
May we honor our stories, support one another, and thrive side by side.
For the women who came before me,
The women standing beside me,
And the women yet to walk this path …
May we rise, strong and radiant.

About the Author

Luci Harrison is a holistic lifestyle coach, certified nutritionist, Pilates instructor, and personal trainer with over fifteen years of experience specializing in midlife. She thrives on helping women feel strong, balanced, and energized through the menopausal transition. As the owner of her own boutique Pilates studio, she's passionate about blending the latest research with real-life practicality. Luci combines medical science with evidence-based strategies and heartfelt coaching to guide others with clarity and confidence.

When she's not coaching or teaching, you'll find her in her garden, painting, capturing beauty through photography, walking in nature with her beloved Aussie Terrier, Baxter, practicing Pilates for core strength, balance and flexibility, or lifting weights to stay strong and grounded.

Synopsis

Welcome to *Your Menopause Balance: a practical, empowering, and deeply personal guide to navigating midlife with strength, clarity, and purpose.* This book is for every woman who has ever wondered "what's happening to me?" and dares to believe there must be more than just surviving.

Drawing from my journey through burnout, hypothyroidism, chronic fatigue, and perimenopause, as well as years of experience as a Pilates teacher, personal trainer, and nutrition coach working with hundreds of women navigating midlife, this book offers the roadmap I wish I ha~~ ~~ blends the latest science with real-world strategies and lived wisdom help you understand your body, balance your hormones, and rebuild you energy from the inside out.

My guide covers the topics that matter most: nutrition that supports midlife metabolism, movement that builds strength without burnout, a focus on gut health, cultivating connection and purpose to bring meaning and joy to this stage of life, and so much more. Your time of "just coping" is over! This book is chock-full of highly valuable and empowering information. Let's uncover the strongest, most radiant version of you. Your midlife crisis is over; welcome to your second act. Shall we make it bold and meaningful? It's your choice.

Contents

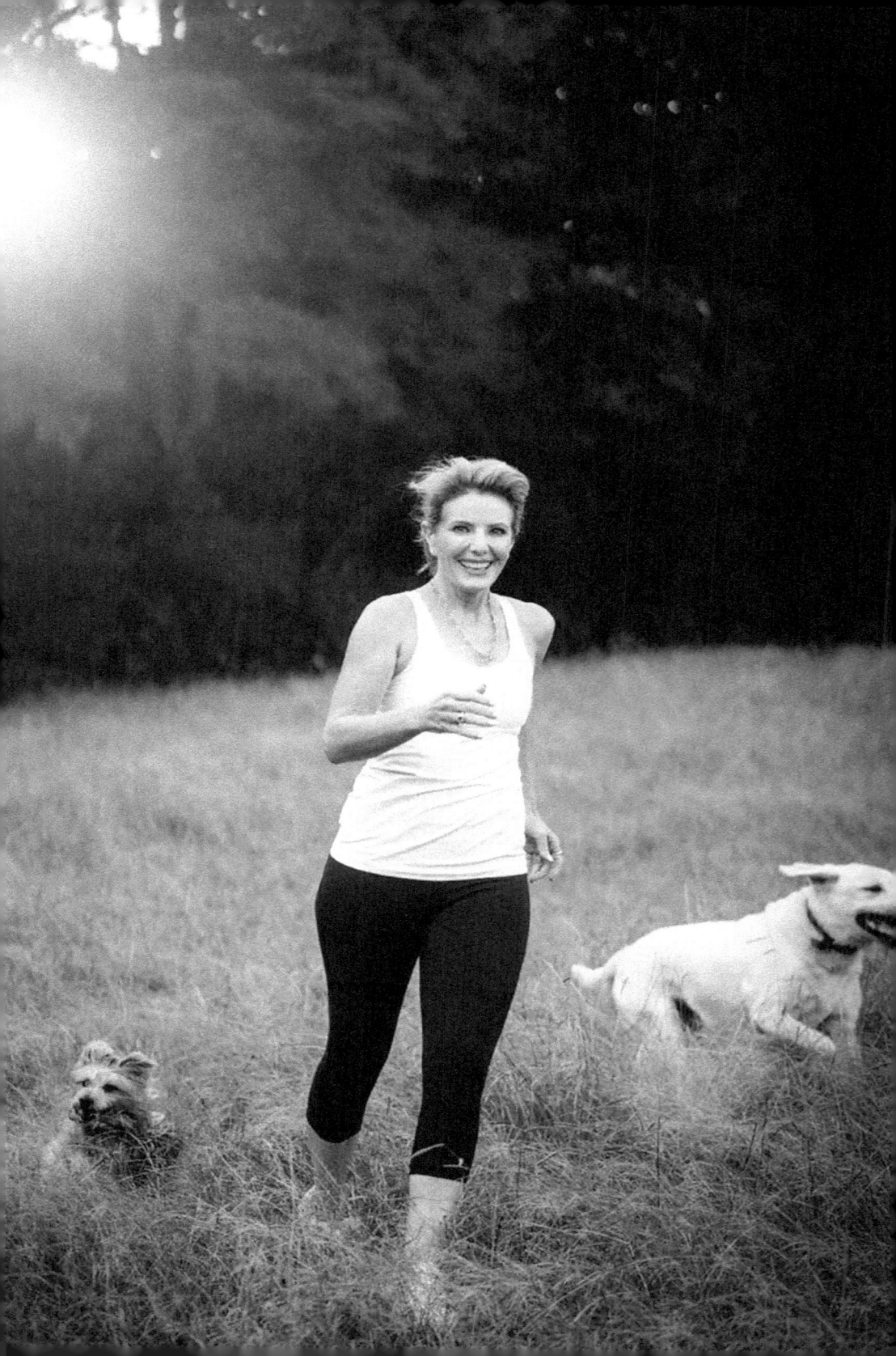

Introduction

Of Farm Life and How Nature Shaped Me

I grew up on a big, wild farm where strength was just how life was lived, not something you worked for. My dad believed in natural resilience. He never set foot in a gym yet looked like a bodybuilder or Tarzan, as we liked to say, especially when he did the farm work in his Speedos (yes, really). His muscles were carved from years of throwing hay bales, chasing cattle on horseback, and wrestling with wire fences (and sometimes us kids). His motto was, "Dads can do anything. And they never, ever give up. There's always another way to get a result." That stuck with me for life.

We were five kids, two boys and three girls, and we all pulled our weight. There were no shortcuts, no pampering, and no 'boy' or 'girl' jobs. Whether it was mending fences, hauling hay, or tending to a sick animal, we were all in it together. It was hard, physical work, and rest days were rare. But there was a profound beauty in that life. I became attuned to the land, the shifting seasons, the moods of the weather and the unspoken language of animals.

I learned early on that nature doesn't wait for you to be ready. If a sick animal lay still too long, we knew it wouldn't make it. So, we'd gently string it up in a supportive harness in the shed and move its legs to get the blood flowing again. We weren't trained vets, but we had grit, compassion, and a surprisingly high tolerance for animal smells. That kind of hands-on, heart-led learning shaped me. It taught me that movement heals, and that care is something you do, not just something you feel. This lesson about the power of movement for a purpose never left me. As Joseph Pilates famously said, "Change happens through movement, and movement heals."

My mum was just as fierce in her own way. She was always on the move, always busy creating. She was passionate about creating magical spaces of color and could often be found in her garden boots, under a big sunhat, tool in one hand, and a grand idea in mind. She added color to every corner around our farmhouse, and somehow, the garden just kept growing—wild, vibrant, and full of life. She showed me that movement could be practical as well as joyful, expressive, and even beautiful. And when she wasn't out in the garden, she'd bring that same vibrant energy to her canvas, painting bold, colorful works of art, or wearing outfits as creative and bright as her personality. Everything she touched told a vivid story.

I was born a chronic asthmatic. From my earliest days, breathing didn't come easily. I spent much of my childhood sick, and I remember moments when simply getting air into my lungs felt like a battle. One of my earliest memories is of my dad driving me up to higher altitudes, softly singing lullabies to calm me down, hoping the elevation and the rhythm of his voice would help me relax enough to breathe. I remember the thick, hot steam baths, too, trying to coax my little lungs open with warmth. When you can't breathe, your whole body goes into panic mode—your chest tightens, your airways clamp down, and it becomes a vicious cycle.

To make things even more interesting, I was also allergic to various substances, including dairy products, animals, pollen, and hay. Not ideal when you're surrounded by all these things as a farm kid. During hay-baling season, while my siblings and cousins were out in the paddock lifting bales, I was plonked into the driver's seat of the big hay truck - even before I could properly see over the wheel. My job, from as young as ten, was to drive slowly through the fields to help the others collect the hay, to keep me away from the thick clouds of dust that instantly set off my asthma.

Often, I could barely reach the pedals, so I'd have to kind of stretch one leg across and lean just right to hit the clutch. And, in my excitement, or panic, to brake quickly when I saw a bale coming, I'd sometimes slam the pedal too hard and send everyone flying. I still remember the day my poor dad flew off the side of the truck like a sack of spuds. No one was hurt (except maybe his ego), but let's say my driving was… memorable. It may have looked like an easy job, but trust me, it was nerve-racking. Still, it gave me a sense of responsibility early on and a real understanding of how to adapt when your body has different needs from everyone else's. Those early experiences taught me resilience, creativity, and that, sometimes, the workarounds we find due to our limitations become the same things that come to shape our strength.

Knocks and Quirks Build Character

Not long after, my own journey with movement took an unexpected turn. In my early teens, I had a bad horseback riding accident that left me with a seriously injured back. Suddenly, all that farm-tough resilience I'd grown up with was no longer enough. I was in pain most days, and my dream of becoming a professional equestrian rider became impossible. That shattered dream was heartbreaking for me as a teenager. It was the kind of loss that leaves a lasting impression.

I also had to find a new way to move that would gently rebuild me. I had to try to focus on the positive, on what I could do, and take small steps to get out of pain, seeking support wherever I could. It wasn't easy, but it taught me the importance of listening to my body, trusting the slower path, and starting again with kindness.

So, while my friends were racing around netball courts or diving off wharves, I was in the pool, doing slow laps, or lying on the floor, learning how to stretch my spine without yelping. That's when I first started exploring beyond the traditional approaches.

I found yoga, acupuncture, osteopaths, meditation, and mindful movement. I learned how to breathe through pain and not to panic, to breathe slow, deep breaths the way I had been taught to do throughout my childhood with asthma. Slowly, I started to listen to my body instead of fighting it. And that shift, that quiet, unexpected detour, became the foundation not just for my healing, but for the entire path that followed.

I didn't move through the education system in the usual way either. School was tough. Back then, no one knew what dyslexia was, so instead of being understood, I was labeled slow or "just not academic." My school career advisor told me I didn't stand a chance of passing school and should probably drop out. But along came Mrs. Ryde, my fierce and fabulous art teacher, who took one look at my work, called it all "a load of codswallop," and handed me the keys to my own art studio. She believed in me when the system didn't. She gave me permission to express the pain I couldn't always put into words through canvas, color, and brushstrokes. That creative freedom became my sanctuary. It was through her encouragement that I found another part of myself. I went on to earn a Bachelor of Fine Arts and later a Master of Fine Arts in photography. I became an international award-winning photographer in my twenties. It was my way of proving them wrong, of saying, "Actually, I am smart enough. I am capable." That fire in my belly to prove I could do anything I set my mind to never left me.

By my thirties, while my friends were running marathons and getting bikini bodies, I was nerding out over fascia, yoga, postural alignment, and how to get someone's core to fire correctly. I trained in Pilates before it was cool, before there were reformer studios on every corner, and before most people even knew how to pronounce transversus abdominis (one of the deep core stabilizers). What began as a workaround for chronic pain evolved into a deep respect for the body's wisdom. My riding accident may have seriously hurt my back, but it gave me the greatest gift of all: the drive to understand movement as medicine, a most powerful tool. And it laid the foundation for the work I now do every single day, which is helping women, especially in midlife, reconnect with their bodies in a way that's kind, sustainable, and strong from the inside out.

Then, Menopause

Twenty years ago, I stood in front of the mirror, a certified Pilates instructor, personal trainer, and holistic lifestyle coach at the peak of physical fitness, thinking I had it all figured out. I owned a little white cottage with a picket fence in a good suburb, something I had worked incredibly hard for and was proud of. I trained intensely, ate clean, juiced regularly, hit the sauna, and pushed my body to its absolute limits, as many of us do in our twenties and thirties, believing we're invincible. I was teaching back-to-back classes. In my "downtime," I swam with the squad, lifted heavy weights, practiced Pilates, and squeezed in hot yoga for good measure. I don't know how or when I managed it, but I was also socializing and trying to start a family. On paper, and even in the mirror, I looked amazing. But was I truly healthy?

When my hormones began to shift around age forty-nine, everything I knew about myself unraveled. My body gave me a clear answer: absolutely not. It was crying out for rest, balance, and compassion. I experienced relentless hot flashes, insomnia, and a constant wired-but-tired feeling. Fatigue consumed me. My digestion slowed to a crawl. Constipation became the norm. My brain felt foggy, and I began forgetting names, appointments, even why I had walked into a room. My body ached, shook, and cramped. My heart raced for no reason. I couldn't tolerate loud noise and was easily overwhelmed. I had restless legs, cold hands and feet, thinning hair, and brittle nails. Sound glamorous? Welcome to perimenopause. Honestly… *what the f*ck was happening to me?*

I hit a wall hard. Bedridden, exhausted, and unable to manage even the simplest tasks. When I tried walking my Labrador, Stan, up a few stairs, I felt like I was carrying a forty-four-pound pack, as well. Finally, at the top, it took ages to catch my breath. I felt deflated. At first, I thought it was the flu. But after a week in bed with no improvement, I dragged myself to my family doctor, who laughed off my symptoms, ran a basic blood test, and said everything was "fine." But I knew, deep in my gut, something was seriously wrong. This wasn't just fatigue. My body felt so depleted that lifting my head or brushing my hair felt like a monumental task. I was no longer functioning. I was barely existing.

Eventually, after months of test after test and trial and error, a hormone specialist diagnosed me with chronic fatigue, hypothyroidism, and full-blown burnout. Oddly enough, I felt relief. I had started to fear something far worse, like cancer. At least now I had names for what I was feeling. And just like that, the high-achieving woman who had built her life around movement, vitality, productivity, and perfectly color-coded to-do lists came crashing down. I couldn't get out of bed, let alone teach a class or tick off tasks. My career, my independence, my identity, everything I had worked so hard to build over thirty years, had vanished in what felt like an instant. It was terrifying.

At first, I didn't know what was happening to me. Then I didn't know how I would survive without work. I'd spent years rushing, ticking off goals, overperforming, saying yes to everything and everyone, proving to the world, and myself, that I was "good enough." I'd pushed my body to its limits in every area of my life.

Sound familiar?

I had built a life that looked "healthy" from the outside, but on the inside, I was running on empty. I learned the hard way, by messing up my own life, failing more times than I can count, and slowly figuring out how to rebuild, piece by piece. I felt like a failure. It seemed like my body had betrayed me. And the worst part? There was no quick fix, no magic solution.

I remember attending a Tony Robbins event years ago. Something he said has always stayed with me: "The number one most important thing in life is your health. Without it, you're no good to yourself or anyone else." That truth hit me hard. Because when your health unravels, everything else does, too. But here's the flipside: When you begin to restore your health, even slowly, everything else will start to rise with it.

This book was born from that breaking point, so that you don't have to reach one to begin healing. I want you to have the roadmap I didn't.

In the years that followed, I dedicated myself to recovery, study, research, and a total realignment. I devoured books, attended every seminar I could find, and worked with a wide range of specialists, including psychologists, to help me cope with the emotional toll. I tried acupuncture, herbal medicine, supplements, medication, and menopausal hormone therapy (MHT). I experimented with countless diets and moved however my body would allow; some days, that meant a slow walk in nature, and other days, it meant lying on my Pilates reformer, gently shifting my arms and legs like a strung-up farm animal (a flashback that made me laugh and cry at the same time).

It wasn't glamorous. It wasn't Instagram-worthy. But it was something. And that something kept me going. Maybe it was having learned to fight as an infant, gasping for breath, or the grit I'd built as a teenager pushing through pain. I just knew I couldn't give up. I had to keep trying, keep searching for anything that might bring a little energy back. And, in time, that approach of doing anything, however tiny, came to save me. These small, slow, consistent actions, done with great care and purpose, changed everything. Not overnight. Not perfectly. But day by day, I rebuilt myself from the inside out.

And now, I get to share what I've learned with you.

What I discovered is that true health, especially in midlife, isn't about pushing harder or doing more. It's about learning to *listen*. Menopause isn't a problem to be fixed. It's a transition to be honored. Your body is no longer a shiny new machine that will run indefinitely on low fuel and no servicing, like it might have in your twenties or thirties. It now needs the same love and attention you'd give to an old friend.

I had to unlearn so much and, at first, these old patterns were tough to change. I let go of punishing workouts that I loved and used to get an adrenaline high from, which were my way of relieving stress but now leave me feeling completely depleted. I embraced movement that felt nourishing instead: walks in nature, strength training designed for a changing body, and Pilates that reconnected me to my core, inside and out. I ditched the rigid food rules I'd been following for years and began listening to what my body truly needed. I adopted an intuitive approach to nourishment, opting for meals that grounded and energized me, free from gluten and dairy. I began replacing the hustle with rest. I built evening rituals, non-negotiable anchors that signaled to my nervous system, *"You're safe now."* No matter how chaotic my day is, I always make space to slow down, breathe, and gently transition into rest.

I also learned to manage stress differently, no longer by trying to control everything but by shifting my mindset. I released what (and who) no longer served me. I stopped chasing the version of me I thought I should be and made space for the woman I was becoming. She was wiser, softer, and even stronger, in a new way. And as I made room for her, my life began to shift with thousands of small, intentional shifts, through my intentional choices.

Guides and Guidance

Years later, when I began coaching women through the entire journey of midlife, from perimenopause to menopause and into postmenopause, I realized just how vital all my earlier lessons had been. Everything I had learned, from pain, slowing down, and listening to what my body truly needed, came flooding back. I saw my clients burning out from overtraining, undereating, overachieving, and pushing through exhaustion, simply because no one had ever shown them how to stop. They didn't know how to listen to their bodies. How to soften rather than harden in the face of difficulty. They felt their bodies were broken. But I knew they weren't at all. They were just imbalanced, just as mine had once been.

I could recognize it instantly: the hunched postures, the forced smiles, the fatigue behind their eyes. I knew that pain, not just physically but also emotionally. I could still feel it in my bones. And instinctively, I knew how to help guide them out of it, one gentle, intentional movement at a time. Midlife turned everything I thought I knew about strength, energy, and wellness on its head. However, it also deepened my purpose and further sharpened my intuition. It helped me show up not only as a teacher but as someone who has been right there.

Now, I'm extending my hand to you. I'm ready to lift you up. And since you're reading my book, you are ready, too!

This book is about relearning the rhythm of your body, letting go of what no longer serves you, and finding your way, through movement, nourishment, rest, and mindset, into a version of midlife that feels grounded, vibrant, and uniquely yours.

Having a mentor who you can relate to, someone who has been there, gone through it all, and come out stronger, can make all the difference.

So, even if I cannot be there with you right now, I hope this book will serve a similar purpose.

One of the most significant mentors in my life was my dear friend Harry. I met him during a gap year in my early twenties. I was working on a ski field and living nearby. Every week, while I was sleeping, a house would arrive across the road as if by magic. Before long, a whole row of homes had popped up. I remember thinking. *How clever. I'd love to meet the person behind this.*

Then, one day, I was sitting at the local pub when a tall, ruggedly handsome man in his fifties walked in. He looked like he'd stepped out of a Wild West movie with gray hair, an oilskin cowboy hat, and a long, weathered coat. That man was Harry.

We started talking and quickly discovered a shared love of art, farming, horseback riding, and property development. I found out he was the one responsible for those relocated homes across from me. He'd recently lost his farm during tough economic times and had to rebuild from scratch. Creating relocatable homes was his way of starting over. A bold, brilliant reinvention.

Harry became a lifelong friend and mentor. He taught me a great deal about courage, thinking outside the box, and not conforming to rules. Like my dad, he believed in never giving up and finding creative ways forward, no matter what life throws at you. Inspired by Harry, I eventually went on to do my share of property developing, buying, renovating, and even relocating houses myself.

Having a mentor like Harry, a wise soul to trust and turn to, has been one of my greatest gifts. He not only carved out new ways ahead, but he also possessed the kind of knowledge and life experience that came from having truly been through it all. He was someone I could trust and often confided in. Over the past thirty-three years, we have shared many adventures. Harry and I had the most honest conversations, too. His support was unwavering.

Although he passed away recently, his positive influence on me remains. To this day, when I encounter a roadblock, I pause and ask,

"What would Harry do?" I still feel like he's right there beside me, quietly guiding me through.

So, I'm not here as a guru. I'm walking beside you, as someone who's cried in doctors' offices and changing rooms, who's tried everything from acupuncture to MHT, and who's come out softer, stronger, and more in tune than ever before. I've lived through the brain fog, the burnout, the confusion, and I've learned that, with the right tools, support, and mindset, it can improve.

I wrote this book in the same spirit: a guide for your undeniably tough time transitioning through midlife. Spoken from my heart, I lovingly assemble tools and plant guideposts throughout, creating a straightforward mentor in paper and ink form for you. I hope that you will take the wisdom within, turn to a new page in your life, and begin to paint in bold, vibrant brushstrokes yourself. Reimagine your future and grow into the person you were always meant to be. Wise, in tune, and utterly in your power. No more playing small or fitting somebody else's idea of who we should be. Together, we shine.

For All of You, Dear Readers

One of the most exhausting chapters of my life was going through a prolonged and ultimately unsuccessful three-year-long IVF journey. The relentless rollercoaster of hope and heartbreak took a toll, not only on my body but also on my sense of self. It also ended my lifelong dream of having a family. Making a bad situation worse, my specialist later linked my IVF hormone treatments to my severe menopause symptoms. Talk about a double blow. Your heart breaks, and then your body pays the price for the hope you held onto so tightly.

If you, too, have walked down the path of fertility treatment and come out the other side empty armed, I see you. The grief is real. And it's vast. And it lingers in the quiet ache of what could have been.

So much of what women carry silently throughout their lives rises to the surface during menopause: invisible grief, pressure to stay positive, thin, pretty, being the perfect partner, and a quiet sense of failure. We go on, creating lives full of meaning, even if they don't look like what we'd imagined. We carry on.

If you, too, have held on tight and built a life or a family of your own design, this book is for you. For the woman who sometimes held on for dear life through the rollercoaster of life and still found a way to keep going. For the woman who didn't get her happily-ever-after but is now reading this book to learn to write a powerful next chapter.

I see you.

Let's rewrite what midlife can feel like together. Right now, it's your moment, where everything can change. It's your season to reclaim your energy. You get to step into your power.

Remember, this book was born from the ashes of my menopause. It's steeped in the real-life stories of many of my clients (which I share on the pages of this book, anonymously). All of them successfully changed their next chapters. Like them, you may soon be another success story.

So, whether you're lost in the fog of your symptoms right now or simply ready to feel more like yourself again, take comfort in this: You're not alone.

I hope this book feels like a hand on your shoulder. A steady, compassionate presence reminding you: You're not broken. You're becoming.

And finally, when I say "woman" in these pages, I'm speaking to everyone who has (had) a womb and experiences the hormonal transitions of menopause. I honor the spectrum of gender identity. Not everyone who navigates this journey identifies as a woman. If you are going through this, this book is for you. You are seen. You are supported.

This book is for all of you.

Let's Explore Together

We'll explore what's happening with your hormones and how to support them naturally. You'll learn how to eat to fuel yourself, improve your sleep, move to feel strong inside and out, and create truly healthy habits that work within the rhythm of your life. We'll explore gut health, hydration for menopause, nervous system regulation, sleep and recovery support, and training strategies. We'll dive into mindset, emotional transitions, and what it truly means to show up for yourself.

You'll learn how to tune in instead of pushing through, how to advocate for yourself at the doctor's office, and how to create rituals that restore rather than deplete you. Because the truth is, you need to begin somewhere, with one small step, one supportive choice, one deeper breath. This book will also provide you with plenty of options and agency.

Not everything in this book will resonate with you, and that's okay. Some things will feel like they were made just for you; others won't. You don't have to take it all on. But I promise you, something will meet you exactly where you are, and that may be just the spark you need.

We live in a world that fears failure. But failure is a wise teacher. Some of my deepest growth came after falling hard, through crash diets, overtraining, and ignoring the signals my body was screaming at me. Those moments were humbling. But they gave me the clarity and resilience to build something far more sustainable. If we reframe failure as a path to self-understanding, it becomes part of the transformation. It shapes us.

This is your chance to rewrite the script. Midlife doesn't have to be a slow unraveling. It can be a fierce reclamation, a time to turn inward, to tune in. You can choose to rebuild your energy, reclaim your joy, and reconnect with the powerful, brilliant woman who has been buried under layers of responsibility, exhaustion, and self-doubt.

This book is here to help you step into a new version of yourself. Not to fix you, but to remind you who you've always been underneath the noise: vibrant, wise, and strong. Let's take this one gentle, doable step at a time. Trust the process. Honor your body. When you care for yourself, you show up stronger for everything and everyone you love.

Let's begin together. Let's step away from outdated stories of decline and into a vibrant new narrative, one of healing, strength, confidence, and clarity. This book is your invitation to come home to your body and your radiant next chapter.

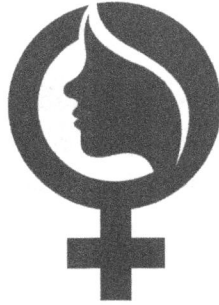

Understanding the Midlife Shift

"So many women I've talked to see menopause as an ending. But I've discovered this is your moment to reinvent yourself after years of focusing on the needs of everyone else. It's your opportunity to get clear about what matters to you and then to pursue that with all your energy, time, and talent."

– OPRAH WINFREY

What an incredible powerhouse of a woman who has reinvented herself time and again! Oprah has experienced profound change and emerged with even greater clarity and focus on her purpose. Her words hit home: this phase of life isn't the end; it's a new beginning.

Midlife doesn't come with a guidebook. One day, you feel on top of things, and the next, your body changes without warning, upending your energy, mood, and sleep. Changing hormones mean what once worked may no longer serve you, and that's okay. We'll reframe this as your invitation to pause, reassess, and realign with who you are today, not who you were a decade ago.

When you begin to understand why your body feels different, you can stop blaming yourself. You can shift from trying to push through to supporting your system instead. This section is about tuning into that shift.

Together, we'll explore what's going on and how to "reinvent yourself," as Oprah puts it. The first step is understanding how we got here. Educated midlife women running successful lives and businesses while caring for their families should know their bodies well enough to navigate this. Or should we?

CHAPTER 1

What Your Hormones are Saying

"Hormones get no respect. We think of them as the elusive chemicals that make us a bit moody, but these magical little molecules do so much more."

– SUSANNAH CAHALAN

This quote sums it up perfectly. Hormones aren't just mood-makers; they're master messengers, influencing everything from energy and sleep to heart, bone, and brain health.

Let's begin with a truth you may already be feeling in your bones: Women's health has been overlooked for generations. For far too long, our worth has been linked to our ability to reproduce. We've been told that fertile looks good. Once that chapter closes, the unspoken message has been that our worth fades away, too, as if wisdom and strength, as well as our life experiences, hold no value.

Even science left us behind. Until recently, most medical research, even for fertility-related treatments, like the pill, was conducted almost entirely on men. Hormonal shifts, and their side effects, and menopause symptoms, simply weren't considered worthy of funding or study. Never mind that they completely rewire us and feel like seismic shifts to our reality. If women complained, their struggles were dismissed as "hysteria," a word that derives from the Greek word for "womb." The implied message: Female troubles are a sissy's complaint. Our wombs were blamed for our frailty and exaggerated suffering. It echoes how women are still too often ignored by their doctors and dismissed as hypochondriacs. No wonder so many of us still carry the sting of being brushed off or told it's all in our heads.

But let's get to the really good and encouraging news: This story is changing.

In the last decade, women's health has finally begun to receive the attention it deserves. We are no longer invisible to researchers, and funding is finally being directed toward exploring women's health. The resulting discoveries are starting to reshape our understanding of menopause. They provide us with a new take on midlife. Our voices are being heard.

Truly, it's hard to fathom how our symptoms were ignored or explained away for so long. But they were. So, it's no wonder many of us feel caught completely off guard when the hot flashes, night sweats, and mood swings arrive. Of course, we're blindsided. No one told us this was coming or how. This was never explained in Biology 101. We hit this midlife like a road bump at full throttle, only to discover we are crashing into a fully-fledged roadblock. What's worse, we have no inkling of how much rest and nourishment our bodies need during this time. That ends here.

From now on, we will talk openly about our hormones. We will claim our shared experiences and discuss them openly. Most importantly, we do finally have the right to give our bodies the care they deserve.

Hormones in Transition

Female reproductive hormones are part of the endocrine system. This network of glands and organs (including adipose tissue) produces and releases hormones.

Hormones carry signals that help maintain the body's balance. These messengers continuously influence your energy levels, metabolism, skin, brain function, sleep patterns, and mood. Like most things in the body, they're always adjusting and adapting to what life throws your way. Sometimes, the messages are clear; sometimes, they can wreak havoc, especially if your body is trying to respond to drastically changing levels.

Progesterone's and Estrogen's Roles in the Body

Let's start with two hormones that have been running the show behind the scenes for most of your life: estrogen and progesterone. Produced mainly in the ovaries during your reproductive years, they're the ones quietly choreographing some of your body's biggest milestones. Think breast development, body curves, and the arrival of your first period. For decades, they keep your cycles turning, support fertility, influence mood, and even shape how you respond to stress. These aren't just "period hormones;" they affect your whole body. When they start to fluctuate wildly at the onset of perimenopause, the ripple effects show up everywhere, from your bones to your brain.

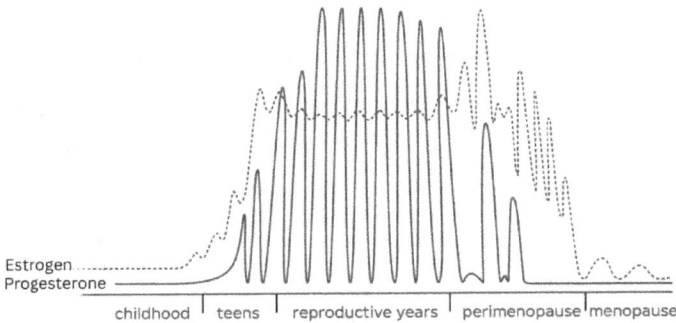

Estrogen .....
Progesterone ——

childhood | teens | reproductive years | perimenopause | menopause

Ovarian hormone fluctuations across a woman's lifespan

Even if your cycle was well-balanced before perimenopause, this can do more than just throw a spinner in the works. It's a hormonal remix reminiscent of the confusing rewiring of puberty (or pregnancy). You may recognize the themes, like amplified puberty blues or hellishly intense PMS on speed. If your cycles were a hormonal rollercoaster before, buckle up! You'll likely be on a wilder ride than you could have ever imagined.

How Estrogen Matters

Estrogen isn't just about reproduction. It's one of your body's star performers, supporting energy, mood, and repair. It keeps your stress response steady, your joints supple, your bones strong, and your brain sharp. It's constantly at work behind the scenes. And here's the kicker:

It's not only about how much estrogen you have, but which type is taking the lead.

Meet the three key players: Estrone (E1), Estradiol (E2), and Estriol (E3). Let's talk about E2 first.

It's the strongest form of estrogen, produced by the ovaries during your reproductive years. E2 is responsible for fertility, conception, pregnancy support, and yes, for keeping sex comfortable by maintaining vaginal tissue thick and elastic, as well as lubricated. As E2 levels decline in perimenopause, things can feel different. Discomfort, dryness, and even pain may appear. Your libido and your sleep take a hit.

This is not just because of E2 levels dropping, but also E1 is ramping up. Where E2 protects, brings down inflammation, and balances your body, the incoming E1 is more like a rogue agent trying to disrupt your peace. Unlike E2, E1 is weaker but can be more inflammatory. Higher body fat and chronic stress can increase E1 production, creating a feedback loop of inflammation, fatigue, and weight gain.

After several years and a full twelve months with no period, you are officially postmenopausal. Hooray? Nope, now your body continues chugging along mostly on E1. The only way to turn the tide around is by addressing your body's signals. And it's a good idea to start sooner rather than later, as there are flow-on effects. Mood swings and anxiety, combined with weight gain, changing body shape, and a knock in confidence can lead to body image struggles and depression.

Bluntly put, there's another major risk: High levels of E1 in postmenopausal women with more body fat are linked to breast cancer and blood clots. If this sounds familiar, it is worth taking action now. Take good care of your long-term health by talking to a health care professional about safe, long-term strategies to reduce risk and support settling at a healthier weight. We will dive into this in more detail in my chapter on weight balance later in the book. For many women, menopausal hormone therapy (MHT) can help restore healthier estrogen levels, especially if started early in this process. MHT can safely top up E2 levels, protecting your bones, brain, heart, and overall quality of life.

It's not a choice driven by vanity. Think of it less as turning back the clock. With a likely lifespan double (if not triple) that of your female ancestors, evolution wasn't counting on us outliving our ovaries by decades! With modern knowledge and care, you can move through this transition with strength, vitality, and balance.

What Progesterone Does

The other female reproductive hormone, progesterone, unsurprisingly, also plays a vital role in various body systems. These include bone, brain, and gum health; mood; muscle and fat tissue; skin elasticity; respiratory and immune functions; cardiovascular health; and kidney function. If you're feeling short of breath, hot, sweaty, and uncomfortable, a change in progesterone levels might be the cause.

Like other sex hormones, progesterone is made from cholesterol and produced by several organs, mostly by the ovaries and placenta, as well as a teeny bit in the adrenal glands. Progesterone is often the first hormone to drop, with perimenopause looming large. Many women don't realize this, but it is often why symptoms begin even while you're still menstruating. This drop can bring irregular cycles, heavier bleeding, migraines, hot flashes, disrupted sleep, and mood swings. It can also lead to so-called "estrogen dominance," which is when estrogen outweighs progesterone, throwing your system even further off balance.

The key is learning to function alongside these changes, even while they're going off like firecrackers. It takes an average of seven years for the menopausal transition from the start of perimenopause to the twelfth month of menopause (the year when your menses came to a full stop). Life postmenopause again requires its own recalibration if you want to thrive.

It's a tough gig, let's be real. If you sometimes feel overwhelmed and at the mercy of your symptoms, you are far from alone. Most women experience symptoms strong enough to impact daily life. Full stop. The severity of symptoms varies from woman to woman and day to day. About one in five reports being severely impacted. Let's call it what it is: Suffering, sometimes debilitating, menopause symptoms that rock your life to its core. If it feels hard to keep up, that's normal. It's not just hormonal. It's a full-body change.

The right help can make a world of difference. From the moment you find a healthcare professional you trust, you're building your support team. My advice: Seek help early and often. If one health care professional dismisses you, get a second opinion (or a third). There's no shame in standing up for yourself and getting answers. If anything, it shows we won't put up with being belittled or put off as hysterical women any longer. Our symptoms are real and demand real answers, real solutions.

And don't be afraid of what you might discover. Armed with knowledge, you become empowered. The more you understand your body, the better equipped you are to support it. Trust me, you have more than just a shot at joy and happiness in your second act.

Menopausal Hormone Therapy

The type and level of estrogen in your body not only keeps things functioning properly but also significantly influences your long-term health. Some cancers, like breast and womb cancer, are affected by estrogen. Factors such as family history, age at menopause, or carrying extra weight can increase the risks. This might sound alarming, but once I understood my risks, I felt a sense of relief. It didn't eliminate the challenges, of course, but knowing my risks gave me the clarity to make informed and empowered choices. I got to decide what was right for my body.

Now, for some more reassuring news: Menopausal hormone therapy (MHT) is now widely accepted as one of the most effective ways to support women through this stage and beyond. For years, hormone replacement therapy (HRT, as it is still referred to by many) had a bad name due to misunderstood and debunked research. Some health professionals may not have kept up with the latest research, but the evidence has definitely moved on. The name change reflects how hormone therapy is now thought of. An essential part of managing menopause. It has nothing to do with fancifully replacing hormones.

I remember how confusing the lack of consensus amongst doctors was to me when I first started looking into hormone therapy. One doctor would warn me off completely, while another explained the newer evidence in a way that finally made sense. That second conversation changed everything. You may encounter similarly confusing, outdated information. Remember, get a second or third opinion. Do not listen to any doctors who say you need to "just ride it out" or the like.

Hormone therapy remains an individual choice. The truth is, though, that when MHT is tailored to you and monitored by a knowledgeable professional, it can be life-changing. It certainly was for me. It did more than just ease my symptoms. It's given me back my energy and clarity, together with my sense of self.

With the right guidance, MHT can ease symptoms and support your long-term health. It lowers several of your risk factors of disease. Essentially, it brings back a lot of the protective effects of the anti-inflammatory estrogen described above, largely without the PMS swings. Depending on when your perimenopause begins, MHT may also play a role in preventing osteoporosis and reducing fracture risk. While the average age of menopause is fifty-one, some women experience it much earlier, whether naturally or due to treatments like chemotherapy.

The latest research shows that starting MHT when symptoms begin may lower your risk of dementia. Researchers now believe there is a "window of opportunity" within the first ten years after menopause when MHT may reduce a lot of the health risks associated with the shift to inflammatory estrogen and lower estrogen levels overall. Catch the window early, and it's like giving your future self a health insurance policy she'll actually thank you for.

When tailored to your needs and monitored with care, MHT can be a powerful supportive tool for thriving in midlife. Almost like bumping into your old self in the mirror and thinking, "Oh, there you are, I've missed you."

CHAPTER 2

Building Your Health Support

"Selfcare is about giving the world the best of you, not what's left of you."

– MARISSA PALMER

Finding the Right Care

For many women, walking into a doctor's office brings more frustration than relief. You explain your symptoms and hope for answers. Then you walk out feeling dismissed, unheard, and without a plan. That's why finding the right care matters so much. You deserve to feel supported and empowered, with treatment options that actually make sense. Too often, women are told, "It's just a natural part of aging." These experiences are far too common and deeply discouraging. No woman should have to convince someone that what she's feeling is real.

Perimenopause often begins in your forties, sometimes earlier. It might sneak in quietly at first: a skipped period here, a restless night there, or that mysterious fog where you forget why you walked into the kitchen. These are your body's gentle nudges that something is shifting. They're important signals; your body is asking for different care. This is not the time to withdraw or dismiss your feelings. It's time to tune in and reach out.

Testing and Tracking What's Really Going On

If you are unsure what you're feeling is the start of perimenopause, a simple blood test can help. The Follicle-Stimulating Hormone (FSH) test can give a snapshot of where you might be in your menopausal transition. While levels can fluctuate, a higher reading may suggest that your ovaries are slowing down and your estrogen and progesterone levels are declining. Because these levels can change from week to week, a single test isn't always conclusive. It's best used alongside your symptoms and medical history, not instead of them. It's not a perfect measure, but it can provide helpful clues and start the conversation with your health care provider about what's really going on.

Talk to your health care provider about whether checking hormones, thyroid function, cortisol, iron, or vitamin levels might be helpful for you. For example, vitamins D and B can decrease with age, and low levels may affect mood, energy, immunity, and bone health. These can offer clues, but no single test tells the whole story.

How you feel day-to-day matters just as much as any number on a page. If your concerns are brushed aside, trust your gut and seek a second opinion. You deserve care that is curious, not dismissive. The right practitioner will take your symptoms seriously and help you explore all options, from lifestyle support to medical treatments.

When Symptoms Don't Make Sense

Changes in hormone levels can lead to a variety of symptoms that show up differently in each of us, making them difficult to diagnose and treat. The list of potential symptoms goes far beyond hot flashes, night sweats, bone loss, or genitourinary changes. You might notice brittle nails and hair, bloating, dry skin, or even strange crawling sensations on the skin. Enough to make you want to pour a glass of wine for relief... and go back for a refill. You're not imagining it. Your symptoms are real and valid. You're not losing your mind; your hormones are just rewriting the script. The list of symptoms is long, and it keeps growing as more research is undertaken on menopause and women's health.

How menopause shows up in your body depends on many factors. Genetics, diet, exercise, stress, smoking, and reproductive history, all play a role. So do body composition, weight, and even cultural beliefs and attitudes toward menopause. Hormonal changes can also reveal underlying conditions that were quietly brewing in the background. Not every woman experiences every symptom, but most notice at least a few, and sometimes it feels like they all arrive at once.

Perimenopause can be unpredictable. It's a time of change and chaos. There's no single blood test that can tell your doctor exactly where you are in the process. Symptoms vary widely, which makes diagnosis tricky. At present, there's also no standard screening for menopause or perimenopause. In medicine, screening helps detect health conditions before symptoms appear. We regularly screen for high blood pressure, certain cancers (like cervical and breast), osteoporosis, and depression. These tools save lives and improve outcomes. While there's not yet a routine screening program for menopause itself, many health checks are recommended during midlife to protect long-term health.

Building Your Support Team

Menopause can't be avoided, but it can be understood and supported. Finding the right help now can empower you to navigate this transition with something resembling grace (or at least fewer meltdowns than a toddler). One of the best first steps is finding a compassionate, informed health care professional who understands perimenopause and takes your symptoms seriously. You want someone on your team who listens, asks questions, and looks at the whole picture—MHT, hormones, nutrition, movement, stress, and sleep. There are no silly questions here.

The best medicine often begins with curiosity. Whether that's your family doctor, integrative practitioner, naturopath, or menopause specialist doesn't matter. You may even build a small team of professionals who each bring a piece of the puzzle. Working with knowledgeable, respectful practitioners gives you back a sense of agency. It's power through partnership and knowledge.

examinations to detect any changes or abnormalities early. Mammograms are the step up and should be scheduled, especially if you are having hormone therapy.

Booking in regular clinical reviews helps to keep an even keel. You know when you'll next get to discuss any symptoms or concerns related to MHT or your overall health. This is your chance to bring up everything. From sleep struggles to brain fog, nothing is too small.

If you want to have the most comprehensive support, ask for the DUTCH (Dried Urine Comprehensive Hormone) test. This test, offered by a company in the USA, measures hormone levels and their ratios in the body. It also assesses whether your liver methylation pathways are working effectively to clear potentially harmful estrogen. It's next level self-care.

Underlying Conditions

If you wake up already exhausted, crash in the afternoon, or need to lie down just to get through dinner, these could be red alerts! Nope, this isn't just age. Yes, you are ageing. You are no longer a spring chicken. But you should have plenty of spring left in your step. These symptoms, especially if persistent, are your body's way of trying to get your attention. It's saying, "I'm overwhelmed. Please help."

What I'm talking about is the kind of tiredness that sleep can't fix. The exhaustion that has settled deep inside you and is changing your life for the worse. Chronic fatigue, burnout, thyroid issues, and other health concerns are often interconnected. And look, while each deserves its own book, they also deserve a mention here, as they often flare up around menopause.

If you're thinking, *"Good god, not more! Stop!"* I totally get it. That's why, for now, let me just drive home that you should not ignore pervasive symptoms. Acceptance is not the answer. Instead, if fatigue or other symptoms persist despite lifestyle changes, lean on your health team and seek a referral to a specialist. Ask questions, request testing, and don't settle for being dismissed. You deserve answers, not shrugs. Stand up for yourself and get to the root of what's going on.

On a side note, I've listed specific conditions, such as chronic fatigue syndrome, thyroid disorders, and autoimmune conditions in the appendix, with short, helpful pointers. For now, hold onto this truth: Seeking help isn't weakness, it's wisdom.

Making It Your Own: Finding What Works for You

Menopause is as individual as your fingerprint. You deserve care that reflects and honors your individuality. Your care team should help you make empowered choices. Standing in your power, you can choose to support your naturally evolving body. This means leaving tried and tested formulas from your thirties behind. Instead, choose to listen to your body's signals. Best to listen before the sirens become deafening, too!

Understanding what's happening behind the scenes, from shifts in hormone levels to changes in stress response, metabolism, and sleep, can be deeply empowering. When you start nourishing yourself, you create a new foundation for your second act. With the right team, a curious mindset, and a little patience, confusion turns into clarity and exhaustion into energy.

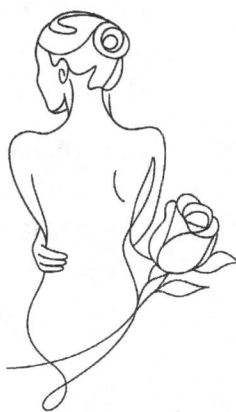

CHAPTER 3

Decoding Your Signals and Symptoms

"Symptoms aren't punishments; they're signals offering insight about what needs care. By listening compassionately, we can begin a healing conversation with ourselves."

– JEFFREY RUTSTEIN, PSYD

Your symptoms are part of your body's well-functioning internal communication system. Listen to your body's whispers. They may feel chaotic, but they carry meaning—all of them. And trust me, there are many, many symptoms of menopause. Thanks to a recent surge in menopause research, we're finally discovering more. We're also uncovering treatment options.

These signals are nudging you to pay attention. They whisper, "Slow down." Though some days, it may feel less like a gentle nudge and more like your body firing off random midnight text alerts: "Hot flash incoming" or "Brain fog loading." When you learn to listen to the signals, they will point you in the right direction. For example, they might be asking you to nourish your nervous system differently. It's time to listen up.

Use your awareness and newfound knowledge to shape your response. With the right approach, your quality of life will lift, and you'll get back into a joyful groove.

And it's not just about how you feel. You'll be proactively lowering your risk of developing worsening symptoms and diseases.

Your body is cleverly communicating. Besides symptoms, you can also find hints in your biomarkers, such as fasting blood sugar, cholesterol, blood pressure, grip strength, bone density, and waist circumference. These give valuable clues. Think of them as your body's dashboard warning lights. You wouldn't ignore the "check engine" light in your car, hoping for the best, would you? Your body deserves the same respect.

Tracking these markers alongside your symptoms is empowering. It helps you and your health care team build a clearer picture of your health. It's about noticing patterns and then making informed, empowering choices.

Are you ready to find out more? Here are some common symptoms and what they're telling you:

Sleep Disruptions: Night Sweats, Wake-ups, and Light Sleep

Hormones play a crucial role in regulating sleep. When hormone levels start shifting, sleep quality can take a serious hit. Progesterone has a calming effect on the brain. It's often called the "relaxation hormone." It promotes deep, restorative sleep.

Estrogen, on the other hand, supports the production and regulation of serotonin. That means it stabilizes mood and the body's sleep-wake hormone, melatonin. As these hormone levels decline, your natural ability to fall asleep, as well as stay asleep, is disrupted. Talk about a double whammy. But it gets worse: low estrogen can impact your body temperature regulation. Say hello to night sweats, another sleep disruptor straight from the hot pits of hell.

It's hard to fathom, but it gets worse: cortisol will rear its head in the very early morning (just what you'd been hoping for). During menopause, these spikes may become further exaggerated due to changes in your glands' comms line, the hypothalamic-pituitary-adrenal (HPA) axis. Cue: sudden wake-ups, early-morning ceiling-staring contests, and difficulty drifting back off.

Sleep is foundational to your health. Your energy, mood, and hormonal balance all depend on it. If you are looking for anything resembling equilibrium, you need those Zs (turn to page 220 to learn how to improve your sleep profoundly).

Solutions:

- Build a wind-down routine to tell your body it's time to rest. Dim the lights, log off screens, and try something calming, like reading, stretching, or gentle breathwork.

- To soothe your nervous system, try legs-up-the-wall, slow breathing, or gentle yoga before bed. This helps reduce cortisol and signals to your body that it's safe to relax.

- Keep your blood sugar steady by eating a protein-rich dinner and avoiding sugary snacks in the evening, which can cause blood sugar crashes and wake-ups during the night.

- Limit caffeine and alcohol before bedtime. Avoid caffeine six to eight hours before bed and skip alcohol at least four hours before sleep. Both disrupt deep, restful sleep, especially during menopause.

- Gently encourage your body into more profound, restorative sleep by using natural sleep-supporting aids, like magnesium glycinate or melatonin, or calming aids like chamomile tea, passionflower, or tart cherry juice.

- Adjust your sleep environment. Swap out synthetic bedding for breathable bamboo or cotton sheets, keep your bedroom cool (ideally, 63 to 66°F or 17 to 19°C), and try using a fan, a cooling pillow, or light layers that you can peel off as needed.

Hot Flashes

Hot flashes can strike like a heat wave out of nowhere, leaving you flushed and drenched. You may also feel pretty agitated, like you've tried a spin class in the sauna. Fluctuating estrogen levels are the culprit, as they affect the thermostat part of your brain, the hypothalamus. Suddenly, it becomes as sensitive to small changes in temperature as a mimosa, overreacting to even the tiniest change in temperature. It thinks you're overheating and rushes to cool you down by dilating blood vessels, spiking heart rate, and sending heat washing over you. Triggers like stress, alcohol, spicy food, or sugar can make symptoms even more intense. Find yourself standing in front of the open freezer? There are some better solutions.

Solutions:

- Dress for cooling. Swap synthetic fabrics (unless they're your favorite sweat-wicking yoga leggings) for breathable, cooling fabrics, like bamboo, linen, and cotton. Wearing loose or layered clothing can also help you respond to sudden inner thermostat malfunctions. Pro tip: Avoid heavy body lotions and use cooling gel-based options instead, if they don't dry out your skin too much.

- Stay hydrated throughout the day, especially with electrolyte-rich drinks, which also help regulate your internal temperature and replenish what's lost through sweating.

- Balance your blood sugar. Avoid refined carbs and sugary snacks, particularly at night. Instead, focus on meals rich in protein, fiber, and healthy fats to stabilize your metabolism and reduce hot flash triggers.

- Reduce triggers. Limit alcohol, caffeine, spicy foods, and hot drinks, especially in the evening.

- Try natural supplements, like black cohosh, sage extract, magnesium, or melatonin. Some women find them helpful in reducing hot flashes.

- Lower your stress levels. When cortisol levels are high, hot flashes often worsen. Carve out moments for breathwork, gentle yoga, meditation, or journaling to cultivate a sense of calm and inner peace. These small rituals can help calm your nervous system and keep you cool from the inside out.

Brain Fog and Memory Lapses

Find yourself weirdly nebulous? Having trouble concentrating? Estrogen loss leads to reduced cerebral glucose metabolism (try saying that three times fast when the brain fog hits, I dare you!). This is essentially a problem getting fuel to areas responsible for memory, decision-making, and verbal fluency. You know the debilitating consequences all too well. It's like running on 1% battery. You feel slow, glitchy, and ready to shut down any moment. You may also notice sugar cravings. That's your brain trying to get a quick fix. Ironically, giving in can spike and crash blood sugar, making the problem even worse.

Lower estrogen also increases neuroinflammation and may impair synaptic plasticity. That makes it harder for the brain to adapt, store, and retrieve information. Hello, wandering around the house asking, "What did I come in here for?" moments.

Finally, declining estrogen levels affect key neurotransmitters essential for learning and memory, including serotonin, which influences mood, focus, and emotional resilience.

Solutions:

- Balance your blood sugar. This means avoiding meal skipping and always pairing carbs with protein, as this helps keep your energy and focus steady.

- Fuel your brain with smart nutrition. Load your plate with omega-3 fatty acids, B vitamins, leafy greens, and foods rich in antioxidants. If brain fog persists, ask your doctor to check key nutrients, such as vitamin B12, D, iron, and thyroid levels—all play a role in mental clarity.

- Move your body daily. Just 20 to 30 minutes of walking, Pilates, or strength training can improve blood flow to your brain and boost clarity. If stress is clouding your thoughts, try breathwork, journaling, or meditation to calm your nervous system and reduce cortisol levels.

- Sleep matters. Your brain processes and resets while you rest, so create a calming bedtime routine and consider magnesium or herbal teas to support deeper sleep.

- Keep your brain engaged. Read, do puzzles, learn something new, or dive into creative projects. Your brain loves a challenge.

Mood Swings and Anxiety

Snapping at your colleagues? Find yourself crying over TV commercials? Forecast: Gloomy with a chance of thunder at best? Fluctuating or declining reproductive hormone levels disrupt the function of neurotransmitters. Without these, emotional regulation becomes about as easy as balancing on a strung-up wire. It makes you vulnerable to anxiety, irritability, restlessness, mood swings, overwhelm, a racing mind, and even depression.

If PMS already hit you hard during your reproductive years, mood stability may seem like a foreign word during perimenopause and menopause.

Solutions:

- Daily movement, whether it's a walk, strength training, Pilates, or even dancing around while vacuuming, helps by naturally boosting your feel-good hormones. Even just 20 minutes can lift a low mood.

- Nourish your brain. Omega-3s from oily fish, chia, or flax help ease inflammation and support emotional stability. Add magnesium-rich foods like leafy greens, nuts, seeds, and be sure to eat protein at every meal to balance blood sugar and stabilize energy and emotions.

- Breathwork and meditation are also powerful tools. Simple practices, such as inhale for 4, hold for 7, exhale for 8 breathing, or taking a few quiet minutes with your eyes closed, can help calm the nervous system and reduce feelings of overwhelm.

- Adaptogenic herbs, like ashwagandha or rhodiola, and magnesium may help build stress resilience if anxiety or mood dips persist. However, always consult a practitioner before adding supplements.

- Reduce alcohol and sugar. They might feel comforting in the short term, but they often worsen anxiety and disrupt hormone balance.

- Sleep is another cornerstone. Create wind-down rituals you love, such as stretching, reading, savoring warm herbal tea, or taking magnesium before bed.

- Tap into the power of connection. Talking to someone who gets it, whether that's a friend, a therapist, or a menopause support group, can bring grounding, perspective, and relief.

- Manage daily stress. Techniques such as yoga, meditation, and deep breathing can help alleviate stress and its impact on hormone levels.

Weight Gain

Hello muffin top! Keeping off the belly weight creep during menopause is no longer "just" about willpower or calories. Hormones, stress, and shifting body chemistry all play a role.

Lower estrogen levels can lead to increased insulin resistance, meaning your blood sugar levels are all over the place. At the same time, cortisol may become the dominant hormone. It's as bad as it sounds: chronically elevated stress hormone levels lovingly encourage fat storage, particularly around the belly. This is more than just a cosmetic concern; belly fat is associated with higher inflammation levels and a higher risk of disease.

Add to that a slowing metabolism courtesy of low estrogen levels. If you don't take action, you may naturally lose muscle mass now. In turn, this lowers your resting calorie burn. Plus, your body may try to hold on to fat cells (fat cells still produce some estrogen—weaker and more inflammatory) as a protective measure. Changing this cycle is about adjusting your approach to match your changing body through nutrition and movement, mostly. If you don't want to end up on a seesaw escalating out of control even while you eat like a bird, it's worth tackling early!

Solutions:

- Strength training is key. Lifting weights or doing resistance-based Pilates helps rebuild lean muscle, which keeps your metabolism humming and supports better blood sugar control.

- Eat enough protein, aiming for 20 to 30 grams per meal, to keep you full, fuel muscle repair, and reduce cravings. Focus on balanced meals with protein, fiber, and healthy fats to steady your energy and avoid sugar crashes.

- Manage stress, as high cortisol levels encourage fat storage, especially around the belly. Walking, deep breathing, yoga, or even just taking ten minutes to pause can help regulate your nervous system.

- Prioritize sleep. It's just as important as food and exercise to avoid sudden weight gain. Poor sleep disrupts the hormones that control hunger and fullness, making it harder to maintain a healthy weight.

- Cut back on alcohol, as it acts like sugar in the body and can stall fat loss. Also, cut sugary drinks, including those that may contain hidden sugar. When eating out, specify "no added sugar" for smoothies or fresh-pressed juices.

- Move more overall. Gentle, consistent movement, especially after meals, improves insulin sensitivity and supports fat burning. A gentle nature walk can do the trick.

- If you have a significant amount of weight to lose, you might also want to find a support system or community, somewhere you feel encouraged, not judged. Having people who get it can make a huge difference in staying motivated.

Fluid Retention

That puffy feeling in your face, ankles, or fingers? It's not your imagination. Fluid retention is a common and frustrating symptom during this shift. Yep, it's the fluctuating hormone levels again. Can you see why I advocate for hormone therapy? Anyhow, hormone changes equal fluid imbalances, making it easier for tissues to retain water.

Low progesterone and high cortisol also affect kidney function and lymphatic drainage, slowing your ability to flush out the excess fluid. Cue swollen ankles, bloating, or tight rings that no longer fit as they once did. Ironically, drinking less or using caffeine as a diuretic may have the opposite effect.

Solutions:
- Support your lymphatic flow. Dry brushing, bouncing gently on a mini rebounder, or taking daily walks can help encourage movement and reduce puffiness. Regular lymphatic massages and infrared saunas can also help support circulation, reduce fluid retention, and promote detoxification.

- Drink more water, even if it sounds counterintuitive. Staying hydrated helps flush excess fluid, especially if you add a squeeze of lemon or a pinch of sea salt to support cellular hydration.

- Take a look at your sodium intake, especially from processed and packaged foods, which are often loaded with hidden salt. Instead, choose fresh, whole foods and season with care. Potassium-rich foods, such as bananas, avocados, leafy greens, and sweet potatoes, help balance out sodium and reduce swelling.

- Monitor your stress levels. High cortisol levels can contribute to fluid retention, so managing stress through breathwork, movement, and regular downtime is equally important.

- Cut back on alcohol and excess caffeine, as they can disrupt fluid balance and stress your kidneys.

- Elevate your legs in the evening, as it can help reduce swelling and support circulation, especially after a long day on your feet. Pro tip: Wear compression socks and leggings whenever possible to help prevent swelling in your lower extremities throughout the day.

Joint Pain and Muscle Aches

If your joints feel, hm, kind of creaky when you get out of bed, or if you're suddenly sore after workouts that used to feel easy, it's not "just old age." Let that old chestnut burn! Joint stiffness and muscle aches are common menopausal symptoms, alongside slower recovery, but that may pale in comparison to the aches and pains.

Your body is missing estrogen's powerful anti-inflammatory properties. Its support of collagen production is also fading. This means joints and connective tissue need help to stay strong, supple, and resilient.

More inflammation also creates greater oxidative stress, adding to the strain on your joints, muscles, and ability to recover.

If getting out of bed is accompanied by snap, crackle, pop, you need to switch up movement, nourishment, hydration, and rest. After all, feeling mobile and pain-free are non-negotiables to enjoy your second act.

Solutions:

- Move your body gently and consistently. Daily movement, like walking, Pilates, mobility exercises, or low-impact strength training, helps lubricate joints and reduce stiffness.

- Nourish your body from the inside out with anti-inflammatory foods, such as omega-3-rich fish, flaxseeds, chia seeds, turmeric, berries, leafy greens, and herbs like ginger.

- Reduce sugar, alcohol, and highly processed foods that fuel inflammation.

- Support collagen production. Try collagen peptides, vitamin C, bone broth, and don't forget adequate protein, which helps repair tissue and maintain muscle mass.

- Hydration plays a surprisingly significant role in joint and muscle comfort. Aim for at least 1.5 to 2 liters of water daily and add electrolytes if you're active or sweating.

- Magnesium is your best friend. It helps ease muscle tension and promote relaxation. Magnesium glycinate or topical magnesium can work wonders on sore areas.

- Incorporate gentle stretching or foam rolling, especially in the morning or after movement, to keep tissues supple and joints mobile.

- Regular massage, infrared saunas, and ice bathing can help soothe sore muscles, reduce inflammation, and relieve the general aches and pains.

- Rest is just as important as movement. Listen to your body and give it the downtime it needs to repair.

Bone and Muscle Loss

As hormone levels decline, you'll naturally lose skeletal muscle. This reduces your body's ability to burn fat. It also leads to increased inflammation. Low estrogen levels increase the risk of osteoporosis. It means your bones are more susceptible to fractures. The combination of a slow loss of muscle and bone leads to frailty as we age.

The good news is it's somewhat preventable and reversible, at least to a degree. Movement and nutrition can safeguard you, together with estrogen therapy. With the right mix of strength training, protein, and smart support, you can reinforce the structure and slow or even prevent muscle and bone loss.

Solutions:

- Regular exercise should include weight-bearing and resistance training to protect your bone health. Include walking, hiking, dancing, and stair climbing to strengthen bones and improve balance, and use weights or resistance bands to build muscle mass. These support bone health and help prevent falls. Just make sure you build slowly. You want to help your body, not inflame or break it down further.

- Nourish your bones with a diet rich in calcium and vitamin D from dairy products, leafy greens, fatty fish, egg yolks, or supplements.

- Sunlight exposure is crucial for vitamin D. Balance this with your need to prevent skin cancer by aiming to expose as much skin as possible for a decent amount of time each day but stay well clear of allowing it to burn. Aim for 10 to 30 minutes a day, depending on your skin type, location, and season.

- Limiting alcohol consumption can help reduce the risk of osteoporosis by improving bone health. Alcohol interferes with the body's ability to absorb essential nutrients vital for maintaining strong bones. Heavy drinking can also impair the function of bone-forming cells and increase the activity of bone-resorbing cells, leading to lower bone density and increased fracture risk.

- Maintaining a healthy weight is crucial for reducing the risk of osteoporosis. Being underweight can lead to lower bone mass and increased fracture risk, while obesity may increase the risk of falls, which can also lead to fractures.

- Quit smoking, as it hurts both bone health and cardiovascular health.

- If you're at a higher risk of osteoporosis, for example, due to early-onset perimenopause, regular bone density scans (DEXA) can help detect early bone loss. There are medications available to slow bone loss and reduce your fracture risk. Speak to your health care professional if you are concerned that you may be at a higher risk.

Changes in Skin

Estrogen stimulates the production of hyaluronic acid, which helps the skin retain and restore moisture; collagen gives the skin strength and structure; and elastin provides elasticity and helps it bounce back into shape. As we live longer and spend more of these years postmenopausal, this spells bad news for our skin.

Some of the most apparent signs of aging are highly visible on our skin: wrinkles, pigmentation, and sagging. Studies have shown that up to 30% of skin collagen can be lost in the first five years after menopause, with an additional two percent loss per year thereafter. If that wasn't shocking enough, it gets worse.

Similarly, skin thickness decreases by about one percent per year. Estrogen therapy can help slow or even partly reverse these changes, supporting thicker, smoother, and more hydrated skin and promoting wound healing by preventing oxidative stress and inflammation. Think of it as nature's own moisturizer running a little low on stock. With the right support, your skin doesn't have to feel tired and crumpled; it can bounce back with a bit more glow, like it's had a good night's sleep (even if you haven't). There is also a range of other helpful tools.

Solutions:

- Hydration is key. Drinking plenty of water helps prevent dry, flaky, and itchy skin from the inside out. Also, remember to have a little salt and an electrolyte-rich fluid.

- Nourishing with water-rich fruit and vegetables, as well as foods high in antioxidants, omega-3 fatty acids, and vitamins A, C, and E will also help your skin bounce back. Eat the rainbow!

- External hydration through moisturizers with hyaluronic acid, ceramides, and glycerin can help draw moisture into the skin. Vitamin C serums help brighten skin, support collagen, and protect against daily environmental stress. Some serums and oils can further boost hydration and improve skin elasticity. You could also opt for non-foaming cleansers or emollient cleansers to avoid stripping your skin of its natural oils. Consider mild exfoliation to remove dead skin cells and promote cell turnover but avoid harsh scrubs.

- Retinoid creams under the guidance of a dermatologist are ideal. They help stimulate collagen production, increase cell turnover, and reduce the appearance of fine lines and wrinkles. They also help unclog pores, reverse some of the damage by fading hyperpigmentation, and improve skin texture. You'll thank yourself later when your skin feels renewed and radiant.

- Daily sunscreen should be part of your morning routine. Make it a broad-spectrum sunscreen with SPF 30 or higher, even on cloudy days. This includes when you sit near a window, as some harmful rays can pass through. Remember to reapply sunscreen every two hours, especially when outdoors.

- Protect the delicate skin on your face, neck, and chest. Hats and sunglasses give extra protection from sun damage.

- Stress and a lack of sleep can increase the number of free radicals aging your skin further (that's not to mention furrows from frowning). Practicing stress-reducing techniques, such as yoga and meditation, can be helpful.

- Regular exercise improves circulation and boosts skin health. Just remember to gently clean away any dirt afterward.

- Maintaining a healthy weight can help your skin appear plumper. Crash dieting is awful, as it not only reduces adipose tissue suddenly but also deprives your skin of vital nutrients.

- Quit smoking now, if you haven't yet. It ages your skin prematurely.

Digestive System Changes

Feeling six months pregnant or experiencing phantom pains in your belly? Sluggish digestion or newly found (yay!) food sensitivities could be the culprits. Estrogen and progesterone both influence your gut. They interact with the enteric nervous system (your "second brain") and gut bacteria. This can hijack your second brain, with effects ranging from lower nutrient absorption to motility issues and inflammation.

Low estrogen has also been linked to "leaky gut" and shifts in microbiome diversity. Do you think this could be behind your food intolerances and IBS-like symptoms? Some days, it can feel like your gut has become an overzealous food critic, sending complaints about everything you eat. The good news? With the right support, you can calm the commentary.

Solutions:

- Slow down at mealtimes. Chewing your food thoroughly and avoiding multitasking helps activate your digestive enzymes, easing the burden on your gut and reducing bloating.

- Gentle daily movement, such as walking, stretching, or even twisting exercises, helps support gut motility, and staying hydrated ensures things keep moving smoothly.

- Support your digestion naturally by boosting stomach acid with a bit of apple cider vinegar in water or sipping warm lemon water before meals.

- Bitter greens, like arugula or dandelion, can also help get digestive juices flowing.

- Add fiber, but gradually. Too much too fast can cause discomfort. Foods like chia seeds, flaxseeds, oats, and a variety of colorful vegetables are excellent choices, especially when paired with sufficient water.

- Add a probiotic, particularly strains like Lactobacillus and Bifidobacterium, or incorporate fermented foods like kefir, sauerkraut, or yogurt (if tolerated).

- Pay attention to everyday gut disruptors, such as sugar, alcohol, fried foods, and ultra-processed meals, which can all throw off your digestive balance.

- Listen to your body. If something leaves you feeling bloated, foggy, or fatigued, it's trying to tell you something.

- Tune into the connection between your gut and your emotions. The gut is susceptible to stress, and practices such as breathwork, meditation, or taking a slow walk after meals can help calm the nervous system and support better digestion.

Heart Palpitations and Anxiety

If you've felt your heart flutter, pound, or race lately, and for no apparent reason, you're not imagining it. It can be alarming and confusing. You may also feel a wave of anxiety wash over you. But there's a perfectly natural explanation: What feels like panic, or a racing heart, is often your body reacting to hormone changes.

Estrogen helps maintain heart rate variability (HRV) and regulates the sympathetic nervous system (your fight-or-flight response). When estrogen falls, HRV decreases, and you may be pushed into fight-or-flight more readily. It can feel a bit like your heart has signed up for an impromptu cardio class (with a dash of panic) without consulting the rest of you. Estrogen's protective effect on the heart is also waning. This heightens your risk of heart disease and stroke. However, there are ways to improve heart health.

Solutions:

- Breathwork is one of the simplest and most effective tools. Deep, slow breathing helps regulate the vagus nerve and calm your nervous system. Techniques like box breathing or inhale for a count of 4 seconds, hold for 7 seconds, exhale for 8 seconds can help reduce the surges of adrenaline that cause your heart to race.

- Keep a trigger journal. Palpitations are commonly linked to caffeine, sugar, alcohol, or emotional stress, and noticing patterns can help you make small but impactful shifts.

- Support your hormones naturally. Foods like flaxseeds, soy, and leafy greens support estrogen metabolism.

- Cardiovascular health matters, as well. Gentle exercise, such as walking, swimming, or cycling, strengthens your heart and helps reduce anxiety. But high-intensity workouts may need to be scaled back if they worsen symptoms.

- Magnesium can be a powerful aid, especially in forms like magnesium glycinate or magnesium taurate, which support both heart rhythm and calmness.

- Stay on top of electrolytes, such as potassium and sodium, if you're active or sweating excessively.

- Create a wind-down ritual to tackle nighttime palpitations. Ditch the screens before bed and try stretching, journaling, or listening to a calming meditation.

- Hydration matters. Dehydration can place extra stress on your cardiovascular system, so aim for at least 1.5 to 2 liters of water a day, more in hot weather or after exercise.

- Speak to your doctor if your palpitations are severe or persistent. Blood tests, ECG, or thyroid checks can rule out any underlying issues.

- Give up smoking. It hurts cardiovascular health.

Vaginal and Urinary Changes

As estrogen levels decline, the health of your entire genitourinary system becomes more fragile. The tissues forming your vulva, vagina, bladder, and urethra can become thinner, drier, and prone to irritation. This can result in everything from itching or burning to urinary urgency, frequent UTIs, and painful sex. It can feel like your body has suddenly rewritten the user manual without telling you.

These changes go by the fun name of genitourinary syndrome of menopause (GSM). It's a common yet underdiagnosed and undertreated condition. Time to get informed and advocate for yourself. Estrogen loss impacts collagen, blood flow, pH, and lubrication of vaginal tissues, so there's zero to be ashamed of. With the right support, comfort and pleasure are absolutely back on the table. When we treat this part of our health with the same attentive care we give to the rest of our body, we reclaim a missing piece of ourselves. Yes, you are allowed to experience pleasure, and most definitely shouldn't be in pain "down there."

Solutions:

- Local low-dose hormone therapy, such as vaginal estrogen (to restore hydration, elasticity, and healthy tissue), is the gold standard for treating genitourinary symptoms. These therapies come as creams, tablets, or vaginal rings, and can significantly improve both vaginal and urinary health.

- Testosterone therapy, often prescribed as a topical cream or gel and used under medical supervision, can be an effective tool to restore desire and improve sexual satisfaction.

- Non-hormonal support, such as hyaluronic acid-based moisturizers, is a gentle natural option. These over-the-counter products provide soothing hydration and help repair delicate tissues.

- Avoid harsh soaps, bubble baths, or scented products that can disrupt your natural pH balance. Stick to gentle, pH-balanced cleansers or just warm water.

- Support your vaginal and urinary microbiome. Incorporating oral or vaginal probiotics, fiber-rich foods, and fermented options like sauerkraut or kefir can help prevent irritation and UTIs.

- Staying sexually active, if desired, while counterintuitive, can support vaginal health by increasing blood flow and tissue elasticity. A good-quality, natural lubricant can make all the difference.

- Nurture emotional intimacy, communication, and self-compassion. Sometimes, low libido isn't just physical; it's emotional, too. Stress, poor sleep, and a disconnect can all impact desire.

- Check the basics. Hydration and urinating after sex help reduce the risk of UTIs and keep everything functioning smoothly.

Tune in, Track, Respond, and Change

Let's put it all to the test. Are you ready? The information I've given you is only worth as much as your willingness to implement the learnings. This is about getting curious, trying out some possible solutions. So, instead of ignoring or battling your symptoms, I invite you to listen to them. Get really curious. Look at every hot flash, brain fog episode, and sleepless night as your body's way of saying, "Hey, I need a little extra support here."

Here's where to start: Tune into your energy. It may feel uncomfortable. Perhaps even downright miserable at first. That's why you're reading this book, right?

Find a moment to notice your body's connection to the ground (through feet, hips, or back). Next, become aware of your breath. Soften your jaw, neck, and shoulders. Allow your breath to rise and fall. Perhaps it will slow naturally, or you could try a breathing technique.

If you can't settle, maybe it's time to move instead! Pop on a song and dance. You could also stretch it out or go for a walk around the block. It often doesn't take much to break through.

You just need to take the first step and let it flow from there. You could place some Post-it notes in a few key areas around the house to remind you to take a quick break. Near your fridge, TV, and even the bathroom are excellent spots. Once you break through a tough moment a couple of times, it gets easier, promise.

When you stop and choose to address your symptoms, you show your body that you are listening. Gradually, your body will respond. You'll build momentum. Keep implementing the simple building blocks progressively and over time, and you'll soon start noticing an upward trend. Keep your eyes on that.

The new you won't be built in a few days (and a few bad days don't mean it's all coming crashing down). Just keep your eyes lifted. Notice those days when you feel better. Soon, they will stretch out, and you will become stronger. Maybe you'll even feel, dare we hope, unstoppable.

On other days, you may still crave stillness or just need a gentle yoga stretch. Taking care of yourself means honoring both types of days. This stage of life is about partnership with yourself. It may take practice, so take it one day at a time.

Please, when the symptoms hit (and they will continue to do so on occasion), remember this is in no way your body failing you. It's speaking up. Think of it this way: Your body isn't staging a revolt; it's sending you little memos. Sometimes, the memo says "rest," sometimes "hydrate," and sometimes "move." When you respond with kindness instead of frustration, you're well on your way.

Symptom Journal

Tracking your symptoms is key. Keeping a journal can be an empowering practice. It doesn't need to be complex. You can just jot down what you're feeling whenever you remember. Jot down any possible triggers you can think of. Over time, patterns emerge, and that noted-down reflection becomes a goldmine of insight. It's fantastic for your supportive health practitioner, too. Think of it as detective work, minus the trench coat; you're simply gathering clues about what your body is trying to tell you.

While there's no universal map for midlife, this will help you chart your course. For example, I learned that a fun night out with a couple of vinos often meant paying a steep price later. There'd be hot flashes, sleeplessness, 3 a.m. ceiling-staring contests, and next-day brain fog and regret. Of course, it was directly related to my indulgence the previous evening. So, ask yourself honestly, "What's keeping me up at night?" Perhaps you may need to forgo the second or third glass to enjoy your next day.

In the chapters ahead, we'll explore practical, real-world strategies to help you navigate these symptoms, step by step. We'll also develop a comprehensive strategy over time. The goal is to enjoy the journey into the new you a little bit. We're not aiming to eliminate every uncomfortable moment. This is about learning to tap into your body's innate wisdom. Let's keep going. You've got this.

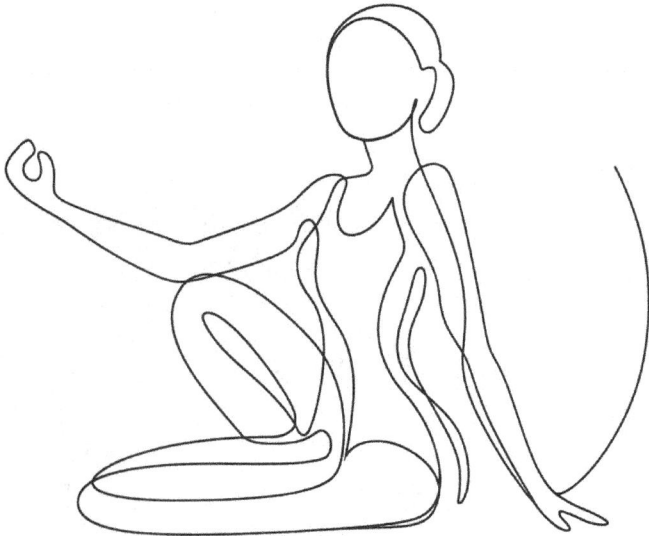

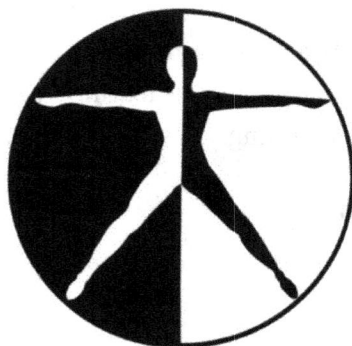

Your Vitality Blueprint

"I see menopause as the start of the next fabulous phase of life as a woman. Now is a time to 'tune in' to our bodies and embrace this new chapter. If anything, I feel more myself and love my body more now, at 58 years old, than ever before."

– KIM CATTRALL, ACTRESS

I love this quote because it challenges the traditional narrative of menopause. Instead of seeing it as something to survive, it encourages us to lean in.

Speaking of assessing honestly what our bodies need: If you're in perimenopause or beyond, you've likely experienced moments, or even whole months, when you felt drained of energy. Perhaps you tried all your usual fixes: trying to exercise more, eat better, and stay productive. Chances are, you still ended up dragging yourself across the finish line, utterly exhausted.

Welcome to your vitality blueprint! We're about to kick-start your cellular engines. Building on a solid foundation of five pillars, we'll get you back up and running. First, let's explore how these engines work.

CHAPTER 4

Energy at a Cellular Level

*"Cellular energy is the foundation of your overall
wellbeing. When your mitochondria are thriving, you'll feel
more energized, mentally sharp, and physically strong.*

— TIME HEALTH

Mitochondria, Hormones, and Circadian Rhythm

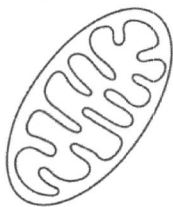

Your mitochondria are tiny structures found in nearly every cell in your body. They're tiny little motors whose primary function is to use nutrients to produce adenosine triphosphate (ATP), the energy currency your body uses for everything from muscle contractions to brain activity. During menopause, declining estrogen levels can impact mitochondrial efficiency. When your cells aren't firing correctly, everything from your clarity and focus to mood and recovery can take a hit.

As estrogen levels begin to fluctuate and decline, your energy production takes a noticeable hit. This happens because estrogen plays a crucial role in how your cells generate energy, regulate blood sugar levels, and maintain a healthy metabolism. Plus, your circadian rhythm, which governs sleep, digestion, hormone release, and energy levels, becomes more sensitive at this stage, compounding the effects. It's no wonder you feel scattered and out of sync (to say the least). Studies show mitochondrial efficiency can drop by up to 30% during menopause.

Let's call these menopausal energy leaks, which come on top of an already accumulated energy debt. Let's not sugarcoat it, most of us haven't exactly lived a Gwyneth Paltrow-esque wellness-focused life until this point, right? Many of us carry a massive energy deficit into menopause already. If you're fighting an uphill battle between commitments and exhaustion, just to then be hit by menopause… hallelujah! Forget about your engine, the wheels are probably about to come off. Signs of persistent energy leaks are poor sleep quality, overworked adrenal glands, nutrient deficiencies, and chronic stress and anxiety. And that's just a small overview.

I discovered this during my crash-and-burn phase. As you may recall, I transitioned from draining myself with intense workouts, running a business, and keeping pace with a demanding schedule to barely making it through a Pilates class without needing to sit down. I wasn't just tired; I was depleted in a way I'd never experienced before. One of my clients, Sarah, a powerhouse CEO, put it best when she said, "It's like someone unplugged half my batteries overnight."

The excellent news is that mitochondria multiply when you stimulate them right. You can boost their energy capacity and resilience simply by moving more. This means challenging yourself with strength training. Granted, it may not be the first thing you feel like doing when the couch is calling loud and clear, but lifting weights sends a powerful message to your body: "We need more energy!" In response, your body gets to work by stimulating mitochondrial growth to meet the increased demand. New mitochondria mean higher energy output, enhanced endurance, and greater resilience. Use it or lose it. Simple.

Challenge your body the right way, and you stop just surviving day to day. Instead, you'll be powering through them like your body just discovered a secret stash of backup chargers.

Take Sharon, a long-time client and former marathon runner turned high-stress executive. When she came to me, she was completely burned out. She was running daily, skipping meals, and living on triple-shot coffees. She joked that her veins were probably 80% caffeine at that point. She was doing everything she thought that would give her energy. Instead, she felt worse: stubborn belly fat, mood swings, insomnia, and constant fatigue. So, we did something radical. We slowed her down. We rebuilt her routine around strength training, Pilates, and just two to three short runs a week. Within weeks, her energy shifted. She could finish her day feeling grounded, connected, and present.

Circadian Rhythm's Impact

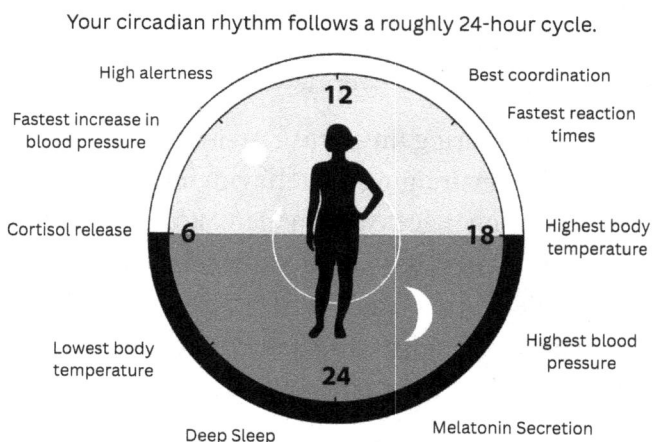

Your circadian rhythm follows a roughly 24-hour cycle.

High alertness

Best coordination

Fastest increase in blood pressure

Fastest reaction times

Cortisol release

Highest body temperature

Lowest body temperature

Highest blood pressure

Deep Sleep

Melatonin Secretion

This internal 24-hour cycle controls many biological functions, including sleep, hormone production, digestion, body temperature, and cell repair. Normally, it's regulated by your brain's response to light and dark. If it gets out of sync, you get knocked off balance. This brings more hot flashes, poor sleep, brain fog, and fatigue. If your internal clock gets thrown, whether due to shift work, artificial light at night, or long-standing habits that don't align with your natural rhythm, it can make everything feel more challenging. I'm looking at you if you're a bit of a night owl. Sleep and steady energy levels may become even more elusive for you during menopause.

You don't have to turn into an early bird, but good habits can work wonders. Restoring a strong day and night rhythm can make all the difference. Light exposure, regular routines, and good sleep hygiene are powerful tools. Think of your circadian rhythm as your body's bossy PA: it likes schedules, hates surprises, and will have a meltdown (in the form of hot flashes and brain fog) if you keep ignoring it. Better work with it: Get morning light, maintain regular mealtimes, and establish sleep rituals. Yes, it may sound boring, but it'll help keep the intercom from buzzing. Your energy levels depend fair and square on your circadian rhythm and your mitochondria. Keep the tiny engines and your bossy PA happy, and you'll reap the rewards.

Repairing Your Energy Grid

Restoring and recharging your internal energy system requires simple, actionable strategies. The right kind of support equals more energy.

Our bodies, including our mitochondria, are highly adaptable. Although menopause throws them off-kilter, they remain highly responsive to small, supportive lifestyle changes. Small, intentional shifts can produce significant results.

I'll never forget one of my lowest moments during perimenopause. It was 3 a.m., and I was standing in my kitchen, drenched in sweat, disoriented, and feeling like a stranger in my own body. I had always been the Energizer Bunny, running a studio, training clients, lifting weights, swimming laps, managing a B&B, and juggling a to-do list most people would find exhausting. Then, suddenly, I could no longer do any of it. I felt foggy, drained, and overwhelmed by even the smallest decisions: what to eat, what to wear, when to move.

One morning, after another night of broken sleep and an intense swim session, I was so depleted I had to sit on a Swiss ball while teaching Pilates. I couldn't even stand up. Soon after, I became too exhausted to lift my head off the pillow. I had to step away from the clients I'd been coaching for years, not because I didn't care, but because I didn't have any answers to my sudden malaise. I was scared. My body was shutting down. My mind felt like it was spiraling out of control.

That was my rock bottom. But it was also the beginning of everything changing. I stopped seeing my symptoms as flaws and started seeing them as signals. It was less like my body was breaking down and more like it was waving a white flag, begging me to call a truce and finally listen. My body had been pleading for support for a long time, and I was finally ready to listen.

I began journaling my energy patterns and adjusting my food and movement based on how I felt, not what I thought I should do. I replaced punishing workouts with restorative ones. I began treating myself with the same compassion I'd been offering to others.

Enduring Energy: Addressing Leaks and Debt

Diving deeper into a supportive mindset, we need to take a moment to step back and reflect on our approach. Making habit changes takes courage. They are also most effective and lasting when broken into manageable steps. We need to introduce them in small, bite-sized portions so you can process them. No need to add to the overwhelm caused by your symptoms. Think of it less as a crash renovation and more as a gentle home makeover, one drawer, one corner, one habit at a time. When executed correctly, this method can make all the difference.

In my own life and working with hundreds of midlife women, I've seen how impactful even the smallest foundational habit changes can be. Maintaining consistent mealtimes and a regular sleep routine helps regulate our circadian rhythm, which in turn supports mitochondrial performance. Gentle, regular movement, especially outdoors, boosts energy production. Irregular eating, chronic stress exposure, and poor sleep habits are like leaving the lights on all night. Eventually, the energy bill comes due.

Nourish, In All Ways

I learned this the hard way. During my go, go, go years, I powered through afternoon slumps with strong coffee and sheer willpower. Spoiler: Willpower is not a food group. It left me wired, exhausted, and struggling to get through the evening. It wasn't until I started respecting my natural rhythms by eating a high-protein, balanced lunch and taking a short rest in the afternoon that I began to recharge sustainably.

Everything changed when I shifted from just "eating light" to genuinely focusing on eating right to nourish my cells. Ironically, I needed more, not less. I stopped random smoothies and squeezing meals in whenever I had time, and instead started choosing intentional meals. I changed my eating habits and prioritized all the good stuff: protein, healthy fats, fiber, and a variety of vibrant, colorful foods. Buh-bye cravings. See you later, empty tank! I also let go of long cardio workouts that left me drained and began choosing movement that supported my nervous system, built strength, and increased my energy. Most importantly, I started treating rest as essential, not as a luxury, but as medicine.

This shift in focus created flow-on effects I would never have dreamed of. Instead of chasing energy spikes followed by crashes, I found a natural cadence, and so did my clients. One woman said, "It's like I've finally found the groove I've been missing for years." We weren't supporting our mitochondrial health before. Now, we regained our natural energy. The physical shift brought mental and emotional improvements, as well.

This isn't about chasing the energy of your thirties. It's about learning how to care for the woman you are now. Work with your body's evolving energy architecture, not against it. If you've been feeling like your batteries are stuck at 10%, know this: It's not about doing more. I know I said you need to challenge your mitochondria, but it's mostly about doing things differently, smartly. Your body will respond eagerly when you meet its needs.

Supporting Your Cells' Engines

As the way you eat, move, rest, and manage stress directly shapes how well your mitochondrial cell engines run, let's look at what this means on a practical level during midlife. Nutrition, stress management, and movement are so much more than just wellness buzzwords; they are the fuel, the maintenance, and the driving style your body relies on.

Think of your body as a vehicle. Your mitochondrial engines need:

- Quality fuel. Nutrient-dense, whole foods supply the raw materials your cells need to produce energy efficiently. Protein, healthy fats, antioxidants, omega-3s, and colorful plants act like premium gasoline, fueling your engine without clogging the system. Slow-burning carbohydrates, such as sweet potatoes, quinoa, lentils, rolled oats, and non-starchy vegetables help balance blood sugar, support hormones, and reduce energy crashes.

- Regular maintenance. Just as a car needs oil changes and tune-ups, your body needs consistent rest and recovery to repair, reset, and rebuild. This includes quality sleep, strategic downtime, and stress regulation to keep your systems running smoothly. Deep rest also boosts mitochondrial repair through autophagy, your body's natural cleanup crew.

- Fasting and meal timing. Overnight breaks of twelve to sixteen hours give your body a chance to clear damaged mitochondria and build stronger, more efficient ones. Balanced spacing between meals supports energy stability. Just keep in mind that fasting isn't one-size-fits-all. During menopause, some women may need to shorten fasts to avoid feeling depleted.

- Gentle driving. Your movement matters. Pushing too hard or running on stress hormones is like riding the brakes downhill—you'll burn out fast. Instead, consider low-impact resistance and strength training, walking, Pilates, yoga, or low-impact HIIT. These are forms of movement that build you up, signal your mitochondria to create more energy, and leaves you stronger instead of worn down.

Energy steadies, your mind feels clearer, and that relentless fatigue starts to lift. The magic happens when we stop pushing through and start working with our bodies. Supporting your mitochondria is one of the most impactful ways to reclaim your energy and feel like yourself again, only this time with more wisdom and self-compassion.

The five pillars supporting your vitality blueprint will be key to achieving the above. Before we get to them, let's take a look at common energy leaks. Existing habits taxing you can have a sneaky way of staying under the radar. Let's find them first. We want to make sure we don't rebuild our foundation full of gaps.

Sneaky Energy Thieves

Just like a house loses heat through tiny cracks and drafty windows in winter, our bodies can "leak" precious energy through unnoticed habits. During menopause, when your system is already working overtime to recalibrate, those leaks can leave you feeling flat, even when you're "doing all the right things."

Take my client, Rachel, for example. She was eating well, getting seven to eight hours of sleep, and still dragging herself through each day. When we looked closer, we found energy drains hiding in plain sight: shallow breathing during high-stress Zoom meetings, skipping lunch breaks under harsh fluorescent lights, and late-night scrolling. Each leak seemed small, until you added them up.

Another common culprit is a suboptimal breakfast. I can't count how many women start their day with seemingly "healthy" choices: fruit, cereal out of a box, or toast with jam. However, with shifting hormones, the quick-burn, high-carb, and hidden sugars start to spike blood sugar, leading to a crash mid-morning. Cue fogginess, irritability, and your third coffee by 10 a.m.

One client, Toni, had this exact pattern until we swapped in a protein-rich breakfast with healthy fats and fiber. Her blood sugar and energy levels stayed balanced throughout the day, and the transformation in her focus and vitality was noticeable within a week.

These little, ingrained habits feel so normal that we rarely question them. But once you start identifying your energy leaks, whether that's emotional overextending, irregular meals, or skipping your afternoon walk, you can begin plugging the holes and protecting your vitality. This chapter is about becoming your energy detective. Because once you spot the leaks, you can act. That's when the real magic begins: You'll get back to consistent energy levels!

Spot the Leaks

Stress, especially the low-level, chronic type, can quietly drain your energy throughout the day. During menopause, your ability to handle stress also drops markedly. It's easy to get stuck in a state of high arousal. Keeping a journal will help you identify potential stressors. Often, we don't realize when we enter a stress response, unless we pause and pay attention. That pause is your best defense against a sudden surge of cortisol, which can spike blood sugar, increase inflammation, disrupt sleep, and leave you feeling wired but exhausted.

For example, I've found myself snappy with emails and drained after small conversations before I realized what was going on. It wasn't major drama, thankfully, but there were a lot of subtle signs: I was constantly checking my phone, found myself clenching my jaw, feeling like I had to be "on" all the time. There were multiple energy leaks.

All those small things add up, of course. With decades of energy debt under your belt, there's likely little buffer left. Your body is signaling you to slow down and recalibrate. If you're operating close to overload with no reserve, even small things can tip you over the edge. You'll go from calm and composed to breathing-fury-at-anyone in no time.

Add in the environmental changes you've had to grapple with over the last few decades. Computers and devices are constant companions nowadays. It's like we've forgotten how to turn ourselves off, just like our gadgets. We've turned into hamsters on a wheel, spinning, scrolling, and proud of our endless hustle. Always on, always available.

Watch out, as exposure to blue light after dusk disrupts your circadian rhythm, to boot. Remember how this is an integral part of mitochondrial health and your energy levels? Thankfully, many devices now have settings that allow for nighttime mode. If you absolutely need to use a screen, those geeky-looking blue-light glasses can actually be surprisingly effective. About time we reduced the blue light that interferes with our sleep.

I used to stay up late working on my laptop, thinking I was being productive and getting ahead. In reality, I was hijacking my sleep, disrupting my circadian rhythm, and stressing my mitochondria. My "productive" habit was quietly sabotaging my recovery and leaving me foggy the next day.

Movement can become another unexpected energy leak if approached incorrectly. We've already discussed how vital it is to tune into your body and avoid overexertion. Later in the book, a whole chapter will be devoted to finding an exercise rhythm that aligns with your body's natural patterns and allows for adjustments when needed.

Trust me, I understand the urge to push yourself hard in the gym. I used to be all about "go hard or go home." That approach is like a completely worn-out sock—it has holes. It no longer looks good on you. It's not that less exercise is better, it's that the right kind of exercise, done with intention, makes all the difference. Plus, you need to get the recovery right! Not as easy as it sounds, if you can't get enough shut-eye. But we'll get to that, too.

I spent years doing intense workouts. From long hikes and brutal HIIT classes, to tough boot camps, and nonstop lap swimming and grueling spin classes, I was the queen of toughing it out. But my body kept saying, "No, thanks." The signals were there. I'd finish workouts more exhausted than I began. I wasn't getting the endorphin high anymore, either.

When I shifted from intensity to consistency, I started slowly regaining my moxie. I added strength training, Pilates, and restorative exercises. Gone were my intense cardo sessions, like my spin classes. I opted for shorter, relaxing walks in nature instead. Soon, I started feeling energized instead of drained.

And we simply cannot and should not forget the emotional weight we carry. Women shoulder so much. It can be more than "just" a contributing factor leading to feeling rundown. It can even take you straight to burnout alley. Now is the time to reassess and be honest with yourself about all those sneaky energy leaks, even if you like being the go-to person for everyone around you. Simply learning to acknowledge the load we shoulder and auditing regularly what gives us energy versus what drains us is excellent practice. Voice it. This may help you feel lighter already.

You'll need to learn to be economical with your energy for a little while. Give yourself the space you need to grow into the new you. Learn to say no to what drains you. Your body needs to be put first for a while. You deserve it! A great practice is to hold a regular "energy audit" in your journal: track your energy boosters and leaks, then use those insights to guide your choices.

One client, Carol, a high-school teacher, mom of three teens, and caregiver to aging parents, realized she was pouring all her energy into everyone else. She was leaving no energy for herself. The sandwich years had caught up with her. She still loved caring, of course, but something had to change. She put her well-being back on the list: weekly Pilates, a daily head-clearing walk, and asking her family and support circle for help. Within months, her energy returned, her posture lifted, and she felt unmistakably different, steadier, and brighter. She came back to herself.

Plug Your Energy Leaks

Here's how to go about turning this around. Start with your first energy audit. For one week, track your energy highs and lows. Get curious. What were you doing, eating, or thinking at those times? Look at your sleep, stress, movement, and emotional load. You'll begin spotting patterns you didn't know were there. Common energy drains requiring simple shifts are:

- Skipping meals or snacking on sugary foods → Stabilize blood sugar with regular, protein-rich, nutrient-dense balanced meals, low in sugar and refined or highly processed carbohydrates.

- Scrolling social media in bed → Replace screens with a book or calming bedtime routine or at least change the light setting on your mobile phone. Your phone can survive the night without you; it doesn't need a midnight scroll-a-thon.

- Shallow breathing under stress → Practice belly breathing or try box breathing (inhale for 4, hold for 4, exhale for 4, hold for 4). Set reminders if needed.

- Lack of natural light → Aim for 10 to 20 minutes outside daily, especially in the morning, barefoot, if possible, to ground yourself and reset your circadian rhythm.

- Eating foods that cause bloating/inflammation → Pay attention to how foods feel, not just what's labeled "healthy."

- Overcommitting when your body says no → Set boundaries and give yourself full permission to rest and say no. Remember, "no" is a complete sentence, not a paragraph of excuses.

Creating an energy-friendly lifestyle doesn't mean changing your life all at once. It's about making small, manageable changes. This could be stepping outside with your morning tea, carving out phone-free moments, or opting for a nourishing lunch instead of a quick carb fix. The goal is awareness and harmony, not perfection. This is about you. How you feel. Not what anybody else thinks.

Tune into your frequency. At first, it may be a bit like adjusting a radio dial through static, until you find a clear signal. You'll know it when you feel it.

In my life, fixing these leaks changed everything. Trust me; I had many leaks. I don't push through anymore. I pause, listen, and choose what fills my cup. When my clients do the same, their energy levels often rebound faster than they'd expected. Because when you stop fighting your body and start working with it, midlife becomes not just manageable but empowering.

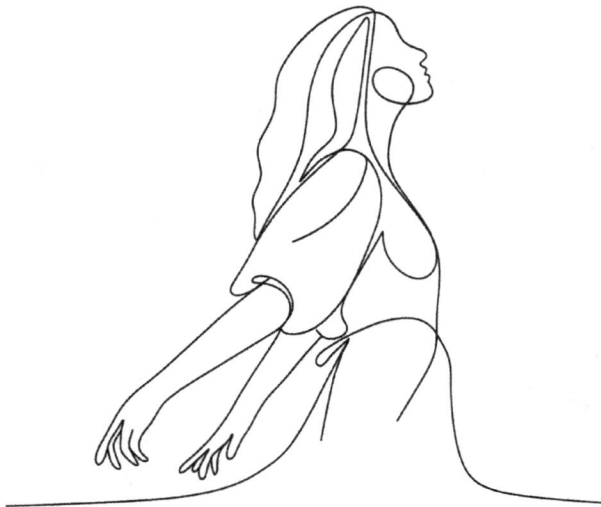

CHAPTER 5

The Five Pillars of Midlife Vitality

"Keep your vitality. A life without health is like a river without water."

– MAXIME LAGACÉ

We've covered how menopause affects your energy system, so now let's explore how to rebuild your energy system in a way that works for you. For your life.

Creating your personal vitality blueprint means finding the right balance for you. A balance that fits your world now. Together, they provide a strong foundation for your new zest in life. Separately, they offer hooks to help you start shifting how you are right now. Grasp onto them, and you'll start shifting your energy levels. You'll build zest back step by step. Your symptom journal can give you an idea of where to start (rather than staring at the whole foundation and feeling overwhelmed). Let's take a look.

Inner Harmony Mindset – Pillar One

Let's discuss emotions for a moment. During perimenopause and menopause, they can suddenly feel like they've been turned up to full volume without warning. One minute, you're okay, and the next, you're crying over a coffee commercial or snapping at someone for breathing too loudly. Sound familiar?

Emotional sensitivity can be one of the earliest signs that your hormones are beginning to shift, even before hot flashes or sleep problems show up. Yet, many women are caught off guard by it. There's a lack of education, so we don't expect to be hit with such drastic biological changes all at once.

This might be one of the most disempowering facts about menopause. You feel like your body is malfunctioning, but you're not encouraged to talk about it. Thankfully, you're reading my book, and I want to tell you: This is normal, too. And it's manageable, changeable.

Midlife can trigger everything from brain fog to anxiety and grief, but it's also a time of remarkable growth and resilience. The Inner Harmony Mindset pillar focuses on emotional intelligence, self-awareness, and self-trust. Because your mindset influences your habits, hormones, and daily energy levels. Managing stress is a vital part of this process.

During perimenopause and menopause, your body becomes more sensitive to stress. You may find that you can't handle it as well as you used to because declining estrogen and progesterone affect your brain's ability to regulate cortisol, your main stress hormone.

You may notice that you don't bounce back from stress the way you did before, and daily challenges can feel more overwhelming. That's not weakness; it's biology. Chronic stress can disrupt your hormones, interfere with sleep, increase inflammation, and leave you feeling wired yet exhausted.

Developing strategies to calm your nervous system as part of the other pillars can make a big difference. This could be breathwork, spending time in nature, or simply making space to rest. Practicing mindfulness, journaling, therapy, or just reframing negative self-talk are also essential tools. They'll help you feel more grounded, clear, and resilient.

Brain health also matters. Keep your mind sharp by learning new things and socializing. I know it may be the opposite of what you feel like doing, but give yourself permission to rest first and invite friends for a cup of tea and a laugh later.

Peter Attia, in his book *Outlive*, highlights how protecting our brain is not only about warding off decline but also about building what he calls a "cognitive reserve." This reserve is like an insurance policy, giving your brain the extra resilience it needs to withstand aging and hormonal shifts. This matters because Alzheimer's and other dementias are now understood to develop decades before symptoms appear.

Engaging your mind regularly will safeguard it. Whether you choose reading or taking up a new hobby, challenge yourself with something that feels a little uncomfortable at first. Just as exercise trains your muscles, novelty and learning train your brain. And it does not have to be complex. Cooking a new recipe, learning a language, or even changing your walking route can spark new neural connections.

Social connections also play a protective role. Conversations with friends, community involvement, or group learning environments provide joy while lowering stress hormones and reducing your risk of cognitive decline.

Movement is brain fuel, too. Exercise improves blood flow, supports mitochondrial function, and encourages the release of the wonderful brain-derived neurotrophic factor (BDNF), which acts like fertilizer for your neurons. Put all the above together, and you'll be tending your inner garden. You'll soon marvel at your brain's flourishing. We'll explore this in depth on page 66.

Quick Tip:

Right now, emotional self-care is an absolute priority. Shift to a self-aware mindset rather than judging or trying to force your way through. I invite you to focus on what's within your control. Go for what you can do without a fight. Breathe. Now gently let go of what is outside of your control. It's not worth your energy. You only have so much energy to give, at least initially. Choose wisely what you spend your precious energy on. Reduce unnecessary chatter, especially when brain fog hits. Your emotional bandwidth is already stretched thin. Practice letting go of distractions, energy drains. If it's not serving you any longer, you don't need it.

Here's how. Say it with me. Pause. Breathe. Ask:

- What energizes me?
- What drains me?
- What do I need more of?
- What can I start saying "no" to?

Keep a simple symptom journal to notice patterns. Practice with an open mind. You'll start to see what truly supports you, and you'll identify what sends you spinning. This knowledge gives you back your power. Seeing the patterns creates greater clarity. And from that clarity, you can create calm and peace. Zen you? Yes, she's within reach.

Nourishing Nutrition – Pillar Two

Food is a powerful form of caring for your body. Every bite you eat helps your body to repair tissues, restore energy, regulate hormones, and protect your long-term health. Good nutrition is essential now. Stat. It heals your body. It's a matter of paying attention now or paying the price in an hour, tomorrow, and the decades yet to come.

When hormones fluctuate and energy levels feel unpredictable, the right nourishment helps you feel grounded. It supports your gut health. You'll have steady blood sugar levels and less inflammation. Your food provides the raw materials your body needs to function optimally. It's time to start thinking of food as nourishment. It'll help you thrive again. Say it with me, "I have permission to nourish my whole body, thoroughly."

Truly nourishing foods have the power to transform how you feel each day, from mood and metabolism to sleep quality, brain function, gut health, and bone strength. Protein helps rebuild and preserve lean muscle. Healthy fats support your brain and hormones. Good-quality carbohydrates provide lasting energy and support serotonin production. Colorful vegetables and fiber-rich foods keep your gut happy and your blood sugar steady. We'll come back to this topic in more detail on page 95.

Midlife isn't the right time to restrict your food intake. Don't deprive your changing body of key nutrients. Instead, it's a truly great time to nourish your body and soul, taking good care of yourself. This often means letting go of outdated beliefs and ingrained ways of responding to our bodies.

As women, our relationships with our bodies are often damaged when we're young. We're taught from an early age that we're judged by how we look. Being slim and svelte is what we're taught to aspire to. Feeling good in our bodies and being powerful doesn't feature much in girls' upbringing. Chasing our dream bodies and viewing our bodies as separate from ourselves does. That's beside the many problems with a lifelong dieting mindset. That approach has to stop at midlife. Your body simply won't cooperate as it did before.

I invite you to reclaim your body fully. Embrace where you are. Now. Be more mindful of how you nourish yourself. Did you read that? Nourish, not just feed or fuel, but truly care for your body. Choose life-affirming, whole, colorful foods. Protein-rich and anti-inflammatory whole foods provide your body with a solid foundation. You're showing yourself care for recalibration and restoration.

When you eat to support your changing body's needs, it'll all get a bit easier. You'll stop just scraping through your days by the skin of your teeth. And you'll be making better, calmer choices. It will become a walk in the park, with a picnic full of delicious, colorful whole foods and in the company of good friends. Visualize it. Choose it.

Quick Tip:

Here's a sneak peek at what this pillar is about. During menopause, your metabolism changes. Weight may be creeping up. This doesn't mean you need less food. You need smarter, more nourishing food. Cut back on processed and sugary foods first. It'll leave you steadier. Build your plate around:

- Protein with every meal, essential for muscle, hormones, and steady blood sugar

- Healthy fats for brain function and hormone production

- Fiber-rich healthy carbs, like leafy greens, colorful vegetables, and legumes to feed your gut and fuel your energy

- Antioxidants to protect your mitochondria from oxidative stress

- Fermented foods or herbs (optional extras to support digestion and microbiome health)

Think: vibrant vegetables, leafy greens, oily fish, avocado, nuts, colorful berries, and plenty of water. Omega-3s are also non-negotiable. I always say, "Every meal is an opportunity to heal or to harm." It doesn't have to be perfect. But let it be intentional.

The Right Movement Choices – Pillar Three

Movement is about learning to speak your body's language. During perimenopause, your nervous system is more sensitive. This means choosing the right type of movement, the right time and duration, and listening to your body's signals. It can (and probably should) also include mindful movement practices. You could give tai chi or yoga a whirl.

Most importantly, it means letting go of the idea of moving to burn calories, chase abs, or impress others. Instead, choose to move in support of yourself. Think of your hormones, muscle mass, posture, bones, brain, and mood. Because the right type of movement and timing can positively impact all of them. Remember, even tiny bits of movement can be powerful. It'll truly transform the way you feel.

But here's the catch: The wrong kind of exercise definitely makes things worse. Unable to focus, losing it at your partner. Long, intense workouts can ramp up menopause symptoms, including fatigue, stubborn weight gain, and sleepless nights. If your adrenals are already taxed, pushing through a tough spin class will rob you of your reserves and might leave you wired, exhausted, or staring at the ceiling instead of sleeping. Instead, your body needs strength-building movement in support of your nervous system.

Let's explore smarter ways to move that work with your hormones. Don't worry; I'm not about to recommend "just" Kegel-type exercises (the classic pelvic floor squeezes you may have heard about). Quite the opposite. Strength training can become your true midlife superpower. It helps maintain lean muscle, supports metabolism, and protects bone density. There's a reason Madonna and other celebrities swear by it when they hit their midlife. Don't worry; we're not aiming to put Arnie to shame. Just regular smart strengthening of your otherwise deteriorating muscles. Frail doesn't have to be your destiny! Strength training doesn't just leave you toned; it can be a fountain of youth. But more on that later.

Combine it with Pilates, yoga, or tai chi. You want nervous system support. On that note, never underestimate the power of a daily walk, especially in the great outdoors. It's free, grounding, and one of the best things you can do for your mood and longevity. All of these are the building blocks of the new you. And, along the way, you'll become strong and flexible. You'll build your body's resilience. You'll lower your risk of disease.

Finally, movement should feel good. It should give you a sense of connection to your body. It's a daily reminder that you're still here, still strong, still vibrant. The right kind of movement reduces stress, releases tension, and improves mood. Whether it's an uplifting Pilates class, a strength training session at the gym, or playing a round of golf with your partner, movement should leave you feeling better than when you started. When you find something you genuinely enjoy, it's not just fitness; it's freedom.

Quick Tip:

Here's something I tell all my clients: Move in ways you enjoy. Don't force yourself onto a treadmill if it makes you miserable. This new approach is about connecting with your body. So, trust your body's wisdom and be kind to yourself. Explore. Play. Dare to try something new.

One of my clients, Anne, in her early fifties, had always dreamed of trying Pilates and golf, but she'd never allowed herself the space to try them. After her children left home, she finally started going to the Pilates studio and the golf course. Just a few months later, she already stood taller and moved with greater ease. She'd decided to do something just for herself, something new, and her posture and confidence showed it. I love seeing this spark in my clients, and I hope you'll be next!

Movement is one of my coaching specialties. Just like nutrition, it plays a vital role in supporting your body beyond menopause. We'll take a deeper dive into it later. You'll learn how movement can help you rebuild strength, support your joints, lift your mood, and boost your energy. If you're ready to start there, feel free to skip ahead. Just remember to revisit the other chapters, as all five pillars are essential for building a strong, healthy postmenopausal life.

Rest and Recovery – Pillar Four

Sleep can sometimes feel like a cruel joke during menopause. One minute, you're yawning and falling asleep at work. The next, you've woken up in the middle of the night with your brain buzzing like you've had a double espresso. Hormonal shifts are the culprits. Add in your fancy new digestive issues, and you've got a real mix of symptoms keeping you awake.

Poor sleep affects your performance and your rest and recovery (vegging out on the couch only counts if you aren't stressing about your to-do list simultaneously). It creates a bit of a vicious cycle.

That foggy-headed, wired-but-tired feeling isn't just an annoying side effect of menopause; it affects everything in your life. What's more, it leads to unhealthy choices. Research shows we give in to cravings and bad habits more when sleep-deprived. Grabbing whatever's in sight during midlife is *not* the answer, even if it may happen (no judgment; been there, done that!). But sleep is a crucial part of midlife wellness. We'll explore this in depth later in the book.

And remember, menopause lowers your stress threshold. Things that used to roll off your back might now feel like personal attacks. That's why calming your nervous system is no longer optional; it's essential (unless running on a short fuse is your idea of fun). The more regulated your system, the easier it gets to shift into rest mode. You will also have fewer thoughts rushing through your head, keeping you awake and interfering with restful sleep. If you can reduce your stress response during the day, especially at bedtime, it can help.

Sleep is your body's opportunity to rebuild. It gets to regulate hormones, rewire your brain, and recharge energy levels (all of which you need more during menopause). Give your body a fighting chance to reset and repair. Your grandma was right; sleep truly is the best medicine. And you deserve it, too.

But rest isn't just what happens overnight. It also means permitting yourself to pause during the day. Say no to things that drain you (remember you're reclaiming your energy!). Lie down for twenty minutes with your eyes closed or take a few slow, mindful breaths to reset your nervous system. There are plenty of ways to calm your system. For now, know that all these small moments add up. Rest isn't a reward for getting everything done. It's one of your most potent tools for balance and vitality.

Quick Tip:

You can't force sleep, but you can invite it. Start by keeping a consistent sleep-wake schedule, even on weekends. Your circadian rhythm loves routine. Set a specific time, then create a soothing wind-down ritual: think soft lighting, herbal tea, a few gentle stretches, and a few minutes of deep breathing. Take care of yourself like you would a child: all gentle, predictable routine to soothe the sugar-craving, anxious-to-wake-in-the-middle-of-the-night you. Put your phone away. Yes, you can do without it, promise. At least use the phone's nighttime function to reduce melatonin-reducing light hitting your brain. Cue your body into rest, not stimulation.

Real rest also means building in recovery pockets: short, intentional moments that down-regulate your nervous system. It might be a ten-minute walk after lunch. Five deep belly breaths between tasks. Legs-up the-wall before dinner. Having a cup of tea without a screen. These small moments are how we "plug in" and recharge throughout the day, not just at bedtime.

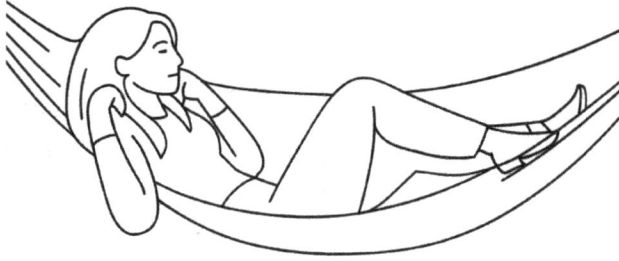

Connection, Joy, and Purpose – Pillar Five

Human connection is a key factor in healthy aging. However, midlife can be unexpectedly lonely for many women, especially those in the "sandwich generation." Simultaneously caring for children, teenagers, and aging parents is taxing. The constant demands can make you feel unseen, exhausted, or detached from yourself and others. There's no time to check in with yourself, let alone friends.

This is precisely the right time to invest in your relationships intentionally. Prioritize regular catch-ups with family and friends, and don't hesitate to seek out new connections. You might join a supportive community, pick up a hobby you've always wanted to try, or enroll in a class that piques your curiosity. Learning something new not only broadens your mind; it also introduces you to people who share your interests.

Whether it's creative expression, spiritual practices, volunteering, or shifting your career to something more aligned, purpose is the fuel that gives meaning to your days. Surround yourself with people who lift you up. Don't underestimate the healing power of laughter, shared meals, or deep conversations. You deserve a meaningful connection, not just with others, but with yourself.

One of the most transformative ways to move forward into your next chapter is by practicing curiosity and wonder, just like children naturally do. I place this pillar last because truly connecting and listening deeply requires feeling calm, present, and able to give freely. It can be challenging to enter this space when you're still dealing with brain fog, constipation, emotional lows, or any of the many other symptoms (though not impossible). You'll find the full chapter on page 254.

But this is most likely the pillar that will have you rejoicing at life and boldly planning your next chapter. So, let's take a look at a few ways to tap into its power.

Quick Tip:

Do you remember that flushed-cheek feeling you get when you're completely absorbed in a favorite hobby? It could be cooking, drawing, fixing your mountain bike, kicking a ball with your grandson, or maybe collecting stamps.

No matter what it is, anything that pulls you into that state is valuable. You want to be so immersed that you forget about time and space. Give yourself plenty of chances to experience this. Arrange exciting or nourishing activities with friends and family, from joining a painting class to an evening at the opera or a hike up a mountain, if you dare (just be sure to leave time to recover!).

When you're going through perimenopausal symptoms, it's all too easy to withdraw, shut down, and turn away from the world. While that has its place, don't let midlife steal your joy. Plan for your symptoms and then enjoy yourself!

Your Vitality Blueprint in Action

You've had a glimpse at the Five Pillars of Midlife Health. Now it's time to weave them into daily life. This is your Vitality Blueprint in action. You'll learn to make small, intentional choices that add up to steady energy, balance, and a renewed sense of self.

Vitality at midlife is less about intensity and more about intention. Don't try to overhaul your whole life overnight; just align slowly. That means starting to adopt simple little habits and rituals to improve your flow. I made quite a few suggestions, but only you know what works for you intuitively. These simple shifts help balance your hormones, boost your energy, and reconnect with yourself. Eventually, you'll find a new rhythm to make your heart sing.

My golden rule is to flex with your flow. This blueprint isn't a rigid schedule. Think of it more as a flexible, evolving flow that allows you to respond to your energy levels each day. Some days, you'll feel strong and clear. Other days, your body might whisper, "Not today." Honor both.

This is about finding flow. Track what fuels you and what drains you with a simple symptom journal. Your body leaves clues every day. Your job is to listen.

Journal Prompt: "What gave me energy today, and what drained it?"

Right now, just acknowledge how you feel. You can respond to what your body is asking for. Give yourself space to process what you've read. Rest, rage, cry, and laugh. Look, you're already practicing kindness and self-care. You're one step closer to getting your mindset into gear.

Think of this process as learning a new language, because you are. You're learning the language of your changing body and emotional landscape. So, just like when you're learning to introduce yourself in French, this is about practice. No one but you cares if you get it right.

It's about redeveloping a learner's mindset and staying connected. Listen to your body and adjust anything you need with care and consideration. Some days, you'll feel like you've got this. Other days... not so much. And that's okay. Learning a new language can sometimes feel overwhelming; that's part of the process.

And you're bound to stumble along the way. But that's okay, too. Failure isn't a flaw; it's feedback. You're learning new ways, and every misstep is just a step toward mastery. So, let's remember: It's gradual progress, laying a foundation for your bright future. Be gentle and compassionate with yourself.

This practice will build your new normal. Caring for yourself wholeheartedly will start feeling so good before you know it. Whether that's a protein-rich lunch, a quiet breathwork moment, or heading to bed fifteen minutes earlier, the momentum builds. It'll propel you toward your goal and keep you going on those days that don't feel so good.

These daily choices may seem minor initially, but together, they add up. They'll lead to your complete transformation. You're not fixing a broken body; you're learning to support a body undergoing an extraordinarily complex and, frankly, awe-inspiring biological rewiring.

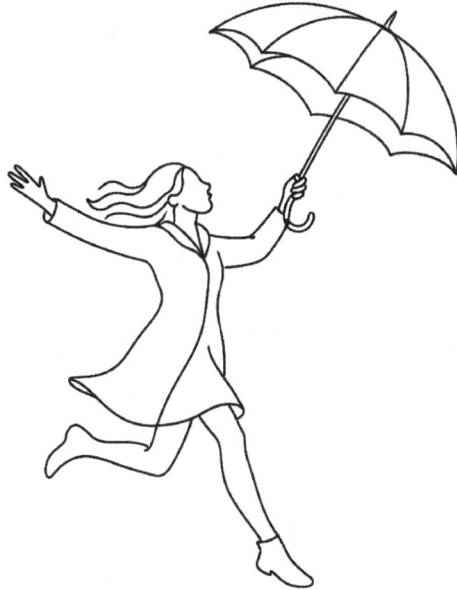

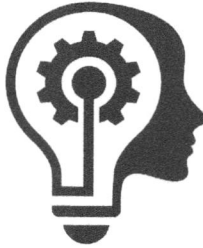

Pillar One – Emotional Wellbeing

"The key to ultimate happiness and fulfillment lies within our own transformation. The more we learn, grow, and evolve as individuals, the more we will find happiness and satisfaction in relationships, work, and life."

– KRISTI BOWMAN

This first pillar is where everything begins. Mindset is the ground you'll stand on as you move through the rest of this book. Without it, even the best nutrition plan, movement routine, or sleep strategy can feel like another burden on an already heavy load. With it, you open yourself to possibility, to curiosity, and to new ways of caring for your body and soul.

Here we lay the foundation for an open mind, one that allows you to learn fresh ways of nourishing your body, discover movement that truly serves you in midlife, reclaim deep and restorative rest, and reignite connection and purpose as you journey toward the spark of your second act.

In the pages ahead, we begin by exploring the inner conversations that shape how you see yourself and your experiences. A shift in perspective can transform challenges into invitations for growth. We also look outward, noticing how the spaces and habits around you either drain your energy or create clarity and calm. By releasing what no longer serves you, you create room for joy, purpose, and the woman you are becoming.

This isn't about perfection. It is about building a compassionate foundation that steadies you as you learn, unlearn, and relearn what truly supports your midlife body and spirit. Think of it as preparing the soil. The other pillars of nourishment, movement, rest, connection, and purpose will take root more deeply when your mindset is open, flexible, and ready. By the time we reach the final pages together, you will see how this inner work paves the way to reigniting your spark for the years ahead.

CHAPTER 6

Inner Harmony Mindset

"Life doesn't end with menopause; it's the beginning of a new adventure. Strap in and enjoy the ride!"

– DAME HELEN MIRREN, ACTRESS

And oh, what a ride it is. Some days, you're unstoppable. Other days, you're crying in the pantry because someone finished the almond butter (possibly you). This rollercoaster is normal when your body, brain, and emotions go through one of the greatest rewiring processes of your life. Think puberty, but with better shoes and more wisdom.

Estrogen is pulling a vanishing act, progesterone is packing up its bags, and cortisol keeps crashing the party uninvited. It's not only reproductive hormones shifting. Stress chemistry shifts, too. These shifts shape your mood, energy, sleep, cravings, and even your patience when someone chews too loudly beside you.

In Traditional Chinese Medicine, menopause is often called "The Second Spring." It isn't seen as a decline but as a time of renewal. Your energy, or Qi, begins to flow differently, moving from reproduction toward creativity, wisdom, and vitality. Once your body no longer uses energy for fertility, it can nourish the heart, mind, and spirit. Menopause is not an ending. It's a beginning. A new season of growth and balance.

Here's the hopeful truth. Your brain can remain highly adaptable, thanks to neuroplasticity. Your mindset doesn't just shape how you think. It changes how you experience menopause itself.

When you stop blaming yourself, you can recognize this as your hormonal reality and begin to support yourself differently. The shift comes when you change the question from "What's wrong with me?" to "What do I need right now?" That one question can turn chaos into compassion.

At midlife, mindset rules everything. It's the first and most powerful Pillar because, without this shift, nothing else truly changes. This season invites reflection and reinvention. What you tell yourself each day quietly shapes the woman you're becoming. And when your inner world steadies, everything else has space to take root and flourish.

Redefining Success and Stress

Stress is a part of life, especially for women juggling everyone else's needs. Left unchecked, stress chips away at both emotional and physical well-being. It fuels anxiety, exhaustion, and that all-too-familiar feeling of running on empty. Many women are so busy caring for others that they don't even realize how much stress has crept into the driver's seat.

Chronic stress is not "just how it is." It drains your body, messes with your hormones, and turns up every menopause symptom: anxiety, mood swings, irritability, brain fog, fatigue, and that deep, quiet pull to retreat for a moment of calm. Left to run the show, it wears you down from the inside out, taking a toll on your heart, gut, immunity, and mood.

According to the American Psychological Association, in 2023, women reported higher stress levels than men. Maybe that's because we are managing families, careers, relationships, and still trying to look like we have it all together.

Then there's the pressure of success. The striving. The overachieving. Add work stress on top of hormonal changes, and you have a recipe for burnout. And let's be honest, it's rarely a graceful topple.

To live the lives we truly want, not just the ones we settle for, we need to redefine success and rethink how we handle stress. True success has room for rest, joy, and connection. If we don't make that shift, the cost to our health, happiness, and peace will only keep rising.

I learned this the hard way. When my eyes were finally forced open, I began living in tune with what truly matters: what my body had been trying to say all along. It all began with a mindset shift.

Again and again, in conversations with clients and friends, the same themes appear. Busyness, overworking, endless scrolling, and under-connecting with ourselves. The spaces that once allowed us to pause and recharge have quietly vanished. There are only so many withdrawals you can make from your health's bank account before you go bankrupt.

There's even a name for the constant rush: "time famine." It's that feeling that there's never enough time for what really matters. You glance at the clock and wonder, "How is it already five o'clock?"

Dr. Seuss said it best:

"How did it get so late so soon?

It's night before it's afternoon.

December is here before it's June.

My goodness, how the time has flewn.

How did it get so late so soon?"

Sound familiar? When we live in constant time famine, we rush past the moments that could restore us.

The truth is, success without space isn't success. It's survival. Midlife is your invitation to stop sprinting and start savoring. Slow the pace. Breathe again. And that's when the transformation begins.

The Midlife Metamorphosis

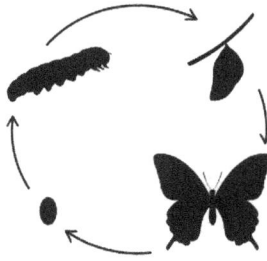

What if midlife isn't a "crisis" but a metamorphosis? Just like a caterpillar in its cocoon, this stage can feel tight and confining: responsibilities pile up, parents age, bodies change, routines start to feel like a burden. But within this cocoon lies the chance for transformation.

This phase invites you to gently reassess what truly matters. Welcome uncertainty as a teacher. Walk forward with curiosity as your guide. Whether it's changing careers, exploring new passions, or redefining relationships, with small steps and steady self-compassion, your second act becomes one of vitality, creativity, and deeply authentic living.

Of course, life at this stage can still feel like standing in the surf, wading through waves of symptoms, curveballs, and the occasional rogue teenager or appliance breakdown. You've already proven you can hold it all together. Now it's about learning to move with life's tides more lightly and more wisely, on your terms.

This means shifting from autopilot to awake. It's realizing that what once worked may no longer serve you. Instead of asking, "What's wrong with me?" try, "What does my body, mind, and soul need right now?" (hint: it's rarely another meeting or family WhatsApp chat).

For years, your worth might have been measured by what you did for others, as a mother, a partner, a colleague, or a caregiver. Now, it's about reclaiming who you are underneath all those roles.

Start small. One shift. One habit. One kind thought. Add another when you're ready. That's how change sticks.

Midlife isn't an ending. It's your creative reboot. You've earned your laugh lines and your boundaries. Now comes the fun part: deciding what comes next.

Know Your Why

Your body is nudging you toward a life that feels more "you." Knowing your "why"–helps you find your path and keeps you moving when motivation runs thin.

Your "why" doesn't have to be grand or dramatic. Maybe it's as simple as waking up feeling good in your skin. Maybe it's about feeling strong enough to chase your grandkids or walk into your sixtieth birthday with pride and sparkle. Perhaps you dream of a second act, running a half marathon, starting a business, or wandering the Camino de Santiago with a backpack and a heart wide open.

Whatever it is, get clear on your "why." Write it down. Say it out loud. Keep it somewhere you'll see when life gets messy: on your mirror, fridge, or phone screen. Include the big, bold dream but also the everyday version. How do you want to feel, and how will you know you're getting there?

Celebrate those small wins: a good night's sleep, a calm mind, jeans that fit comfortably again. They're proof the needle is moving. Over time, those everyday victories add up, helping you stay the course. They'll either hold you back or open the door to growth.

Psychologists call it the difference between a fixed and a growth mindset. I call it flexible thinking for midlife. Less yoga pose, more *life pose*.

The Fixed and the Flexible Midlife Mindset

A fixed mindset whispers, "This is just how I am now. It's too late to change." It interprets hot flashes, weight gain, or brain fog as aging decline, with less vitality, fewer opportunities, and a shrinking world. If you've ever thought, "I'll never feel sexy again," or "There's no point in starting something new at my age," that's your fixed mindset talking. It thrives on fear, comparison, and self-criticism.

A flexible mindset, on the other hand, accepts reality without letting it define you. It sees menopause as a natural transition. Stark and uncomfortable at times, yes, but quietly full of renewal. Setbacks aren't proof you're broken. They're invitations to adapt.

It asks simple but powerful questions:

- What can I learn from this shift?
- How can I grow through it?

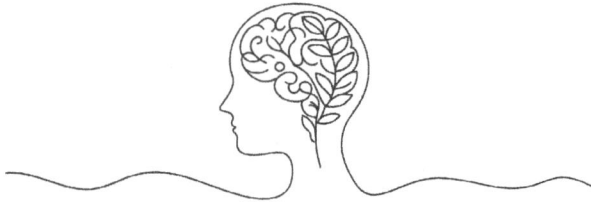

A Simple Reframe

Catch the fixed voice and ask, "How else could I see this?" The magic lies in the reframe. Instead of "I'll never feel strong again," ask, "What's one small step I can take today to rebuild strength?"

- Instead of "My sex life is over," ask, "How might intimacy look different, and even better, for me now?"
- Instead of "I can't learn new things at my age," ask, "What's one skill I'd love to try purely for the joy of it?"

Each small reframe builds a new way of thinking, carving fresh neural pathways that gently guide your brain and body out of survival mode and into possibility and growth. A flexible mindset stays open to learning new ways of thinking and living. It's about curiosity and small shifts that support change. As you read this book, keep that flexibility close. Some ideas may feel new at first. Give them space. Change begins with an open mind and grows quietly into transformation.

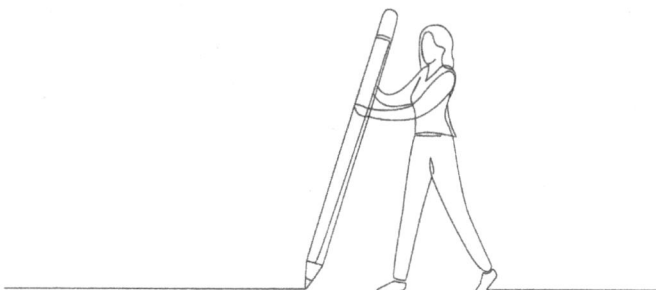

Advocacy and Boundaries

Ask for what you need without guilt or apology. Advocacy is about becoming your own best ally, like pushing for the blood tests you know matter, telling your partner you need a quiet night in instead of another social event, or asking for flexibility at work when symptoms flare.

Boundaries go hand in hand with this. They are gentle fences that protect your energy, your rest, and your well-being. When you respect your limits and voice your needs, you are giving others the chance to meet you where you are. You also remind yourself that your health and happiness matter just as much as anyone else's.

A simple reframe can help. Instead of thinking, "I don't want to be difficult," try, "I am practicing being my own champion."

Mood and Mindset

"Trust your gut" takes on new meaning during menopause. Your belly and your brain talk constantly. When hormones shift, the communication lines between body and mind can get scrambled, like a Wi-Fi signal cutting in and out just when you need it most. Cue brain fog, mood swings, anxiety, or that out-of-nowhere wave of tears. Totally normal. You're not losing it. Your brain's just rewiring.

Tanya, a brilliant university professor, described her brain fog as "thinking through mud." Lectures that once flowed effortlessly became frustrating word-hunts. It wasn't just hormones at play; stress, disrupted sleep, and lifestyle factors were adding fuel to the fog. Once she started adjusting her mindset and daily rhythms, her clarity began to return. So did her spark.

Dr. Lisa Mosconi's groundbreaking book *The XX Brain* is a favorite; it explains how women's brains are uniquely affected by menopause and why they deserve their own science. When estrogen dips, the brain switches fuel sources from glucose to ketones. That can feel like fog, fatigue, or forgetfulness. But the good news is, with the right support, a Mediterranean-style diet, regular movement, deep sleep, and stress care, our brains can still thrive. A happy heart is a happy brain, and blood flow feeds both.

When moods swing wildly, swap blame for curiosity. Ask, "What does my body need right now?" That one question builds self-trust. It reminds you that your emotions aren't betraying you but guiding you.

The Hormone-Mood Connection

At times, it may feel like your emotions are running the show. What's really happening is that your brain chemistry is shifting gears. Your emotional resilience and stress response get tested. This is why you may find yourself more sensitive, reactive, or tearful, even when everything seems "fine."

I'll never forget one afternoon during my perimenopause transition when a speeding ticket tipped me into a full-blown sobbing meltdown. Not because of the fine. It was just the last straw (honestly, Meryl Streep would've applauded the performance). That moment taught me something: my moods are closely linked with my body. The dips often followed a poor night's sleep, a skipped meal, or days of nonstop stress. Sometimes, I craved movement. Other times, my body wanted a nourishing meal. Sometimes, all I needed were stretchy pants, zero social interaction, and a feel-good movie where everything ends well.

Your emotions are simply messages. They're not your enemy. They're gentle (and sometimes dramatic) signals pointing you toward what you truly need: rest, nourishment, support, or just permission to pause. And sometimes, those emotional signals show up on your plate.

Emotional Eating

Emotional eating in midlife isn't a willpower failure. It's biology. As estrogen dips, brain chemicals, like serotonin and dopamine, start to wobble and cravings turn up the volume. Add a rush of cortisol when stress hits, and suddenly a teenager's eye-roll can feel like a crisis that only a bag of chips can fix.

You're not broken. You're human. Your brain is wired to seek comfort. Often, what feels like hunger is really your nervous system calling for calm, safety, rest, or a little kindness. The shift happens when you stop shaming yourself and start pausing with curiosity. I call this the Conscious Pause Point. When your craving hits, take a breath and ask, "What do I need right now?" Sometimes, it really is food. Often, it's something else: a glass of water, a stretch, a laugh with a friend, or simply permission to do absolutely nothing for ten minutes.

If you notice the cookie tin calling, try pairing that urge with a reset. Step outside, sip something warm, or text someone who makes you smile. Even tiny pauses retrain your brain to find comfort in more than one place. Over time, your body learns it has options and that calm doesn't always come wrapped in chocolate. We'll return to these themes later in the book.

Quick Reset Button for a Midlife Meltdown

Sometimes, midlife emotions hit like a storm: fast, fierce, and out of nowhere. One minute, you're fine, and the next, you're snapping over a dishwasher that won't load itself. That's your inner tiger moment. Pause, breathe. It's just asking for a reset. You don't need hours of meditation or a luxury retreat. You need simple tools to calm the chaos in real time, your first-aid kit for the mind.

1. Breathe Before You React

Place your feet flat on the floor. Drop your shoulders. Say to yourself, "I am safe. There is no tiger."

Now, inhale through your nose for four counts, hold for four, and exhale through your mouth for six. Repeat this three times, letting the exhale last a little longer each time. This gentle shift tells your body, "It's okay to relax." I've used it myself, even live on national television, and it saved me from saying something truly ridiculous.

2. Ask a Grounding Question

When doubt or irritation start swirling, pause. Instead of reacting, ask, "What does my body need from me right now?" or "What lesson is this moment offering?" Then add a small physical reset, a sip of water, a stretch, or a step outside. You'll feel your perspective shift almost instantly. Curiosity calms faster than criticism.

3. Flip the Script

Catch one runaway thought and give it a rewrite. Instead of "I can't cope," try, "This moment is hard, but it will pass." If you're blaming someone else, turn it inward with compassion: "What part of this can I take responsibility for right now?" Even a tiny shift from helpless to capable rewires your mood.

Human Being vs. Human Doing

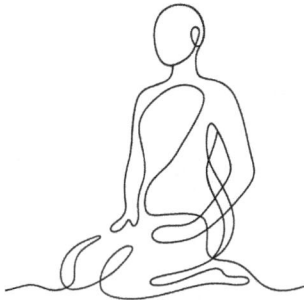

Our culture trains us to measure worth by how much we achieve, tick off, or juggle in a day. That's living as "human doings," our identity gets tangled up in output. We rush from one thing to the next, filling every quiet moment with busyness. But that busyness rarely feels intentional. It's often just a clever way of avoiding stillness or the thoughts that come with it.

Living as a "human being" is different. It's about presence over performance. It's knowing your worth doesn't depend on your to-do list. It's the exhale that comes when you stop proving and start allowing.

A human being can sit in stillness, even for a minute, without reaching for her phone. She gives herself permission to do nothing, to just be. In that space, she starts to remember what actually lights her up.

This season of life invites deeper questions: *Who am I without the roles I play? What am I grateful for? What do I want more of in this next season of life?* You don't need all the answers right away. Just start by slowing down enough to listen. And one of the simplest ways to practice being, not doing, is through meditation.

Meditation Awareness

Meditation has been with me since a horse-riding accident at thirteen. A pain specialist at the hospital taught me to get curious instead of fighting.

Sitting in a quiet, still state, eyes closed, I focused on my breath. "Picture the pain as an eagle's claws gripping your back," she said. "Now imagine those claws slowly unclenching, flying away." Oddly enough, it worked. Something shifted, and I've been meditating ever since.

You don't need mountaintops or mantras. Just a few breaths and a willingness to be still. It's not about escaping your body. It's returning to it with awareness and kindness. That's when your nervous system flips from "fight or flight" to "rest and restore." Breathing slows, cortisol drops, and your body feels safe enough to exhale.

There's no one way to meditate. Follow your breath. Scan your body. Try a guided track. I love Deepak Chopra's reminder: "Holding on is like holding your breath. You will suffocate. Let go." That's meditation: letting go of tension, expectations, and holding it all together. When sitting still feels impossible, take it outside. Slow walking. Breathing. Noticing the ground under your feet. Nature becomes its own kind of meditation, helping you come back to yourself.

For some, meditation is also spiritual. Prayer, reflection, or time spent in a faith community can feel deeply calming. A quiet moment of stillness. A feeling of belonging when life feels uncertain. Lighting a candle, saying a prayer, or simply trusting that something greater is guiding you, spirituality can offer comfort and peace through the waves of menopause.

Meditation hasn't made me perfectly Zen, but it has made me more present, more honest, and better able to pause before reacting, at least some of the time.

If you're new to it, don't overthink it. You don't need incense, crystals, or a guru. Just a few minutes, one breath, and a spot to sit. Meditation is simply the practice of returning to yourself, again and again.

Inner Dialogue

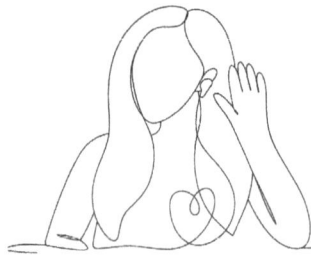

Everyone doubts themselves at times. Everyone wakes in the night and wonders if they're on the right path. That's part of being human. But mindset gives you the resilience to keep going.

We live in a noisy world, bombarded with fear and bad news. But within you is a quieter voice, the one that believes in possibility. Turn that one up. Your mindset is the volume knob.

Negative self-talk raises cortisol levels, turning a small hot flash into a full-body meltdown... and all because someone bought the wrong brand of almond milk. Kind words, on the other hand, calm the nervous system, balance hormones, and help smooth the rough patches of this transition.

Quick reality check: Would you say the things you're saying to yourself to an old friend? If the answer is no, it's time to change your tone.

One tool I love is the Compassion Check-In. It's a reset for when your inner voice is mid-tantrum in the toy aisle of your brain.

- Acknowledge. Name what you're feeling without judgment. It could be: "This is hard," or "I'm feeling overwhelmed."

- Remember. Millions of women are riding this hormonal rollercoaster, too. Some even with their hands in the air screaming, "*Wheee!*"

- Comfort. Place a hand on your heart and say something kind: "I'm doing my best," "This will pass," or "I deserve care and support." And if you feel like adding, "And I'm still a badass," go for it.

- Practice. Rewiring your inner dialogue isn't a one-and-done task, like finally deleting your ex's number (even though, yes, it's time). It's a daily practice, one small, slightly awkward, beautifully human moment at a time.

Especially during symptom surges, on days when hot flashes rage, and when brain fog sets in. These small acts of compassion matter most. Otherwise, your inner dialogue will gleefully grab a megaphone and start shouting.

Here are a few practical ways to help you build emotional resilience:

Five Keys to a Beautiful Midlife Mindset

1. Choose to Tidy Up Your Mind

What you feed your mind shapes how you feel. Be mindful of what you allow in. Notice what you're tuning into, be that endless scrolling or negative news. Turn off phone notifications, skip the gossip magazines, and step away from other people's drama.

When you wake up, resist the urge to reach straight for your phone. Instead, pause, take a breath, and practice daily mindfulness, even if it's

CHAPTER 7

Detox Your Life

"When you live surrounded by clutter, it is impossible to have clarity about what you are doing in your life."

– KAREN KINGSTON

Clear Your Clutter, Clear Your Energy

Decluttering restores clarity, creates ease, and opens space for who you are becoming. Clutter isn't only physical, though; it's mental and emotional, too. The state of our surroundings often mirrors the state of our inner world. Clearing what no longer serves you externally helps shift your thinking internally, which goes back to what we talked about in the mindset chapter.

The truth is, many of us reach midlife with more than a few drawers, wardrobes, or garages filled with items we haven't touched in years. It accumulates gradually: sentimental keepsakes, unfinished projects, clothes we no longer wear, kitchen gadgets still in boxes. All of it carries energy, and that energy can feel heavy.

If you've ever helped a parent downsize or sort through a lifetime of belongings, you'll understand the emotional and physical weight of "stuff." But here's how to reframe: Clearing clutter isn't only downsizing your life; it's lifting the mental fog, reducing decision fatigue, and creating more space to focus on joy, purpose, and what truly matters now. In other words, decluttering your environment helps declutter your mind.

Create Space

A cluttered environment increases mental noise. When you're already dealing with brain fog, mood swings, or low energy, visual clutter only makes it worse. Each drawer you organize, each item you let go of is like giving your nervous system more space to breathe easily.

For me, decluttering has become a personal ritual, a way to reset. I'm talking about small, manageable actions, like tossing expired supplements, unsubscribing from spam emails, editing my wardrobe, and ditching products I'll never use. It's not about minimalism; it's about mindfulness. If something no longer supports the woman you are today, let it go.

Here are a few simple tips to start clearing space.

- Transparent storage boxes. Ideal for pantries, bathroom products, supplements, or seasonal clothes. If you can see it, you'll use it.

- Label everything. It saves you time and mental effort, especially when your memory isn't what it used to be.

- Keep a "donate + release" box visible. Each week, drop in a few items you're ready to let go of.

- Set a 15-minute timer. One drawer. One shelf. One bag of odds and ends. Progress without the overwhelm.

- Ask this powerful question: "Does this still support who I'm becoming?" If the answer's no, thank it and release it.

Remember, this is about allowing yourself to let go of what no longer serves you and creating a space that reflects your current values, lifestyle, and energy.

Your Pantry

One of the most overlooked tools for supporting your health in midlife is your kitchen setup. Your environment influences your choices. And when it comes to food, convenience often wins. Start with a compassionate kitchen audit. What's hiding in your pantry? What food choices are sabotaging your energy, mood, or hormones?

Move tempting snacks, like chips, crackers, and sugary treats, out of reach or completely out of the house. If other family members want them, that's fine; just store them in opaque containers on higher shelves. Please don't keep them in your direct line of sight. Be honest with yourself about your weaknesses. Mine? Chocolate mint cookies. I can open a pack with the best intentions and find half the tray gone in ten minutes.

If there's food that always hijacks your self-control, it's okay to take a break from it. Clearing out doesn't mean saying goodbye to pleasure. You're making space for more intentional joy. When your kitchen supports your well-being, it becomes a space of power, not pressure. Once you've cleaned out your pantry and lightened your toxic load, you'll be ready to set yourself up for nourishing ease.

Batch Cooking

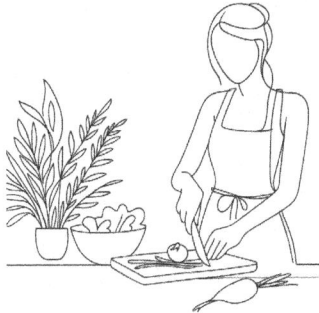

Batch cooking is one of the best gifts you can give your future self. Pick a day (Sunday is always a good choice), and prepare some staples: roasted vegetables, grilled protein, grain bowls, a frittata, or energy balls (protein bites). Store them in labeled glass containers (using a whiteboard marker on the lid works great) so you can see what you have at a glance. When you're exhausted or pressed for time, your fridge becomes a source of calm rather than chaos.

Just prepare enough, so that making good choices becomes easy. Even a few containers of pre-washed greens, chopped fruit, or a batch of homemade soup make a huge difference midweek. Once the clutter is cleared, set yourself up for the week. Batch cooking is convenient and conserves energy. On those "can't be bothered" days (and there will be many), having nutrient-rich meals ready is a lifesaver.

It's the kind of preparation that pays off all week. You'll eat better, feel more organized, and break the cycle of grabbing quick fixes when energy crashes happen. Even if everything else seems chaotic, being prepared helps life run more smoothly.

Clearing the Way Forward

Midlife invites a new rhythm, one that values simplicity and space. Remember, you don't need to do it all in one weekend. One shelf. One snack swap. One drawer at a time. Your energy matters. Your space matters. And you deserve a life, and a home, that feels as clear and powerful as you're becoming.

Let's face it, midlife is full. Full of responsibilities, shifting hormones, fluctuating energy, and often unpredictable days. That's why preparing your meals in advance is a form of self-care. It's about setting up your week with less chaos and more nourishment so that when you hit that tired, overstimulated Wednesday afternoon slump, something satisfying and stabilizing awaits you. Real, grounding food.

It begins with something simple: your storage. Using good containers (glass or BPA-free) makes all the difference. They're more durable, safer for your hormones, and they keep food looking fresh even by day three. It's a small investment that helps your week run smoother and shows care for your future self.

Shopping becomes simpler when you have a plan. Choose a few go-to meals and stock up on staples that nourish you well: colorful vegetables, whole grains, quality proteins, and healthy fats. Just real, nutrient-rich food that makes you feel good.

And while you're planning, take a look beyond your pantry and toward your bathroom shelf. Because what goes on your body is just as important as what goes in it.

Self-Care Swaps

Your skin is your largest organ, and it absorbs more than we often realize. Shampoo, body lotion, deodorant, makeup, and even soap all contribute to your body's chemical load. During menopause, when your hormones are already under stress, even small amounts of hormone-disrupting chemicals can disrupt the balance.

I'll admit, I used to think clean skincare was just a fad. But then I experienced brain fog, forgetfulness (like blanking on my own phone number mid-Pilates class), and a feeling that my system was overwhelmed. That's when I started making small swaps. I switched to aluminum-free deodorant, chose essential oils instead of synthetic fragrances, and used natural products made from vinegar and lemon. Gradually, things changed. My skin felt calmer. My moods stabilized.

Some ingredients to watch out for include parabens (synthetic preservatives that mimic estrogen), phthalates (often hidden under the word "fragrance," which can contain hundreds of unlisted chemicals), and sodium lauryl sulfate (this foaming agent strips your skin of its natural oils). Triclosan is another one to avoid. It's commonly found in antibacterial soaps and has been linked to thyroid disruption. And then there's aluminum, usually found in antiperspirants, a known endocrine disruptor.

Instead, look for products with ingredients you recognize, like coconut oil, aloe vera, shea butter, or jojoba. Choose essential oils over synthetic perfumes. Opt for glass packaging whenever possible, especially for oils and creams. They're affordable and surprisingly effective.

Even small changes, like switching to a magnesium-rich body oil, can help lower your toxin levels. It's like cleaning out your pantry, but for your skin and hormones. One thoughtful change at a time adds up. And your midlife body notices and responds with more calm and, often, more glow.

Cleaning Products

And while we're on the topic of skincare and personal products, there's another sneaky source of hormone disruptors we often overlook: the cleaning products we use at home. What you spray on your kitchen counter or mop onto the floor doesn't stay there. It gets on your skin, into your lungs and, in turn, into your system.

Many commercial cleaners are full of harsh chemicals, artificial scents, and endocrine-disrupting compounds that quietly add to the stress your body is already dealing with during perimenopause and menopause. Your skin absorbs it. You breathe it in. And your body has to process all of it. To clean your home, you can go old-school with vinegar, lemon, and baking soda.

Clear Clutter, Clear Mind

While you're clearing out, don't forget about the clutter in your home environment. I know for me, even an untidy bedroom can leave me feeling scattered and disorganized. When I can't find anything, my already hormonal mind feels even more chaotic. There's a quote I love: "If you want to change the world, start by making your bed." It's often attributed to U.S. Navy Admiral William H. McRaven, who shared it in a commencement speech at the University of Texas. He explained that completing a small task first thing in the morning creates a sense of accomplishment and sets the tone for the rest of your day. And if my bed is made and my room is tidy, I feel more at peace. At the end of a long day, I walk into an uncluttered space that is set up for rest, which helps me reset.

And while we're at it, let's talk about your wardrobe. Your clothes should mirror who you are right now, not who you once were or who you think you should be. Are you still holding onto your nine-inch heels, miniskirts, and low-cut tops from a different era? Or clothes that no longer fit but you've been holding onto for years, hoping they'll fit again someday? Let them go. You'll create space for the woman you are today.

Here's what works for me:

- Group your clothes by category, from shirts to pants to dresses, and then organize by color.

- Shoes go together in pairs, one heel forward and the other toe forward to save space.

- Pop sandals and flip-flops into a small basket or container for easy access.

Here's a fun tip: Invite a trusted girlfriend over, pour a glass of bubbles, and try on every item you own. Sit on the bed, laugh, and create three piles: Yes, No, and Maybe. You'll be amazed at how quickly it all gets sorted. When you clear clutter, each piece you let go of makes space for who you're becoming.

Your Circle Matters

Let's talk about friends and all the people you choose to surround yourself with. The people in your life influence your energy, your confidence, and even your sense of identity. They can either make you feel like you belong, like you're seen and celebrated, or they can make you question yourself. I know this from personal experience.

There was a time in my life when my ex-husband thought my friends were "privileged" and "not normal." Slowly, I became isolated from them. I stopped sharing, stopped showing up, and convinced myself that maybe he was right. But deep down, I missed them terribly. Eventually, I realized that they are and always have been my tribe. They are gold to me. They are like family. These are the women I'd want beside me if the ship went down. We share the same values. We laugh at the same things. We lift each other and remind one another of who we truly are.

Years ago, during a Tony Robbins course, we did a powerful exercise about friendship. We were asked to write down the names of twenty friends on a piece of paper. On another sheet, we drew a horizontal line across the middle to represent the body. Below the line symbolized the gut, above the line, the heart. Then, as each friend's name was read out, we had to notice where we felt them land in our body. Were they in your heart? A pain in your gut? A lump in your throat?

It surprised me. Some names, I expected to feel a connection to, and they didn't. Others stirred feelings of discomfort I hadn't acknowledged. It's a confronting but powerful exercise. What you do with the results is up to you, but it's worth reflecting on, like the clutter in your wardrobe or under your kitchen sink.

It's worth asking:

- Do your friendships reflect who you are today? Or are you holding onto people out of obligation, guilt, or habit?

- Are you showing up for them because you think they need you more than you need them?

Your energy is precious. Surround yourself with people who believe in you and bring out the best in you.

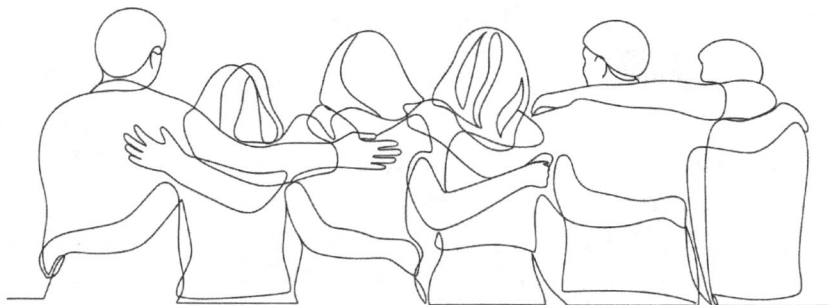

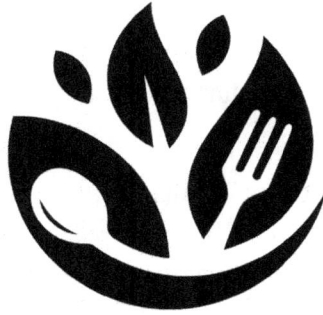

Pillar Two – Nourish to Flourish

"One cannot think well, love well, sleep well, if one has not dined well."

– VIRGINIA WOOLF

How incredible our bodies are, right? They're built to find balance. The moment you start paying attention to their needs, everything begins to shift. Nourish them well with the right combination of healthy, wholesome foods and plenty of water, and they flourish. They're not unlike tiny ecosystems that need a gentle touch when weather patterns shift too much. The moment you tune in and notice signals, you'll see they're all there. And once you gain some momentum, the positive changes begin to happen on their own, triggering a multitude of healthy pathways.

Of course, this might feel a bit different when you're in the kitchen at 3 p.m., bloated like a beach ball, wondering why your digestion now feels like you've had rocks for breakfast and seeing no way out. But here's how to reframe: Midlife is a chance to care for yourself with more knowledge, kindness, and intention than ever before. Your symptoms are signals guiding you. That rock-hard feeling in your gut can be changed. It may not even require much. Start by treating your body gently. Drink chamomile or fennel tea to soothe your stomach. Gently massage your belly in bed. And decide to start your next day gently, even if you're running on little sleep.

Make nourishing choices. Consider protein-rich chia pudding with nuts, seeds, yogurt, and a handful of berries. Move a little while doing the dishes or as you get ready for your day. Play some music to take your mind off last night. Choose to nourish your whole body. We start with life-affirming, joyful nutrition.

In this part, we'll explore the basics of what nourishes your body from the inside out, starting with gut health. We'll also cover hydration, a straightforward look at supplements, and how to balance your weight. It's all about deeply nourishing your body in ways that support your hormones, energy, and vitality so you can thrive.

CHAPTER 8

Gut Harmony

*"Good gut flora has been shown to reduce the prevalence
of allergy and underpin the immune system. They have
potential to be beneficial to human health. Care for your
gut and improve your quality of life."*

– MARLENE HOCHSTRASSER

Your Second Brain

Your gut is a living, breathing ecosystem that influences your hormones, brain, and mood. Think of it as your inner garden. When it's nurtured with the right conditions (hint: not just coffee with a side of panic), it thrives. When it's neglected, things become overgrown quickly.

One of the most important (but often overlooked) connections in this garden is the gut-brain axis, a strong, two-way communication system between your digestive system and your brain. This internal communication network uses nerves (like your built-in calm switch, the vagus nerve), hormones, and immune signals to send continuous feedback, affecting mood, memory, and more.

Hormonal shifts, especially the menopausal decrease in estrogen and progesterone levels, can disrupt this delicate communication system. These hormones play a crucial role in regulating gut motility, maintaining microbiome balance, and controlling inflammation. When they decline, the gut may struggle to function properly, leading to bloating, food sensitivities, sluggish digestion, and irregular bowel habits. Tend to your inner garden, and you tend to your whole self: mind, body, and mood.

During my midlife journey, when I first started experiencing extreme fatigue, it felt as if my entire system had shut down. My belly would swell up like I was six months pregnant, and my digestion would completely stall. It was nothing like I had ever experienced before (my stomach had always been flat). I remember feeling embarrassed about going out. I'd wear oversized coats just to hide my stomach. I was painfully bloated and uncomfortable in my skin.

That was a turning point for me. I realized that supporting my gut health wasn't just a nice-to-have; it was essential for my overall well-being and recovery. Once I started focusing on healing my digestion, everything began to change. Gradually, my energy returned, the bloating eased, and I finally felt like I had some control over my body again.

I first encountered this during Emma's journey in full color. Like many women hitting the menopause speed bump, she got caught in the typical cycle: skipping meals to "get rid of the belly," surviving on lettuce leaves and caffeine, then raiding the fridge like a woman possessed by 9 p.m. Sound familiar? You're not alone. As a holistic and nutrition coach, I see this all the time: women believing they're doing the "right thing" by eating less, only to end up more exhausted, more bloated, and wondering where the hell their energy (and patience) went.

The truth is that menopause is not the time to cut back and punish your body. It's time to fuel your body properly, to nourish it instead of neglecting it. In this chapter, we'll explore how to shift from restriction to true nourishment.

Your Inner Ecosystem

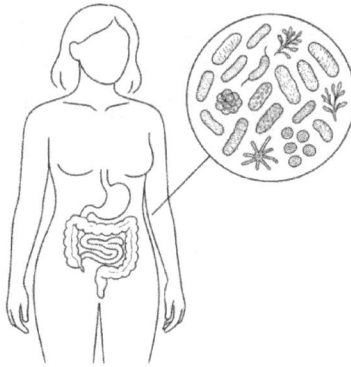

Understanding the complex connection between gut health and hormones is one of my secret tools for thriving during menopause. Think of your gut microbiome as a bustling garden, teeming with life below the surface. Each microbe is like a tiny gardener, tending to balance, resilience, and growth. When this ecosystem is nourished, everything flourishes—from your mood and metabolism to your hormones.

One of the most fascinating recent scientific discoveries (hello, nerdy me) is the discovery of the estrobolome, a group of gut bacteria that help metabolize and regulate your body's estrogen. When these beneficial bacteria are thriving, they help maintain balanced estrogen levels. But when your microbiome gets out of sync (hello, stress, processed foods, antibiotics, and hormonal changes), things can become a bit messy. Too much or too little estrogen can lead to various familiar menopausal symptoms.

During my midlife journey, I learned that supporting these beneficial bacteria isn't just taking a probiotic and hoping for the best. You're creating the right environment so they can thrive, especially when hormones, stress, and sleep disruptions can upset your gut's balance.

That starts with prebiotics, which are types of dietary fiber that feed the friendly bacteria already living in your gut. These foods help the good bugs multiply and outcompete the unhelpful ones. Eating for your gut bacteria helps them grow stronger, become more diverse, and keep that internal garden thriving, boosting digestion, mood, immunity, and hormone balance along the way.

The connection between your gut and hormones is a two-way street. As estrogen levels naturally fluctuate and decline during menopause, they can disturb your gut bacteria balance. When your gut bacteria change, it impacts how well your body processes hormones. It's like a seesaw: if one side goes out of balance, the whole system can wobble.

I've seen this happen many times with my clients. Take Janet, for example. She came to me completely fed up with her severe bloating, low mood, and feeling like her body had turned against her. When we started tracking her symptoms, we noticed a clear pattern: Her digestive issues and mood swings would get worse in sync with her hormonal fluctuations. By focusing on nurturing her gut health through specific foods, daily habits, and stress management, her bloating decreased, her mood stabilized, and she finally felt like herself again.

Happy Gut, Happy Mood

Your gut is your body's second brain. About 90% of your serotonin, the "feel-good" neurotransmitter that regulates mood, sleep, and pain perception, is made in your gut. That's why a happy gut often leads to a happier you. When your microbiome is balanced, you're better able to handle the emotional and physical changes that menopause can bring. Supporting your gut health depends on how you eat, not just what. Speed-eating at your laptop, grabbing bites while driving, or scrolling your phone between mouthfuls (guilty!) can all add extra stress to your digestion. I advise my clients to practice mindful eating. This simply means treating your meals as moments of nourishment rather than another task to rush through.

Try sitting down properly, even if it's just you and your dog giving you judging looks. Set the table and taste your food. Put your knife and fork down between bites. Notice the flavors, textures, and scents. Maybe even take a deep breath or two between mouthfuls. Trust me; your nervous system will thank you.

It's best to aim to spend about twenty minutes enjoying a meal. That gives your brain enough time to receive the "I'm full!" message from your stomach, aiding digestion and reducing those annoying cravings that occur later, especially when we eat too fast and are too distracted. By understanding and honoring the gut-hormone connection, you equip yourself with a powerful tool to navigate menopause with greater ease and comfort.

When you nourish your gut, you're creating a ripple effect that supports hormone balance, mood resilience, energy stability, and overall well-being. And let's be honest, feeling less bloated, more energized, and a whole lot saner is a midlife superpower worth working for.

Healing Your Digestive System

If you feel like your digestive system suddenly became a diva during menopause, you're not alone. Many women notice that their once-reliable digestion starts acting up, making them wonder how they suddenly developed a stomach problem. Let's discuss why these changes happen and, more importantly, how you can restore your balance.

Bloating and Gas

Hormonal changes during menopause can slow digestion and disturb your gut's natural rhythm. The comfort foods you once loved may now feel like you've swallowed a balloon. It may surprise you, but excess air in your abdomen can cause everything from bloating and gas to severe pain and even issues passing your stools (yes, we're going there).

The fix often isn't ditching your favorite foods; it's slowing down, something we have discussed before. Chew properly, avoid chugging water with meals, and try not to eat in a rush or while on the go.

Stress signals can shut down digestion faster than a laptop overheating during a Zoom call. When that happens, your body stops prioritizing rest and digest mode. Eating calmly helps reignite your digestive fire, making your gut's job easier (and your waistband might thank you for it).

Constipation

Not only is constipation uncomfortable, but it's also an added hormonal risk (talk about a double whammy!). When elimination slows down, your body can't effectively remove excess hormones or toxins. This creates a vicious cycle that keeps you stuck, both literally and figuratively. Lower estrogen can also weaken the muscle tone of your gut, making regular bathroom visits feel like a distant dream.

Staying hydrated, especially with warm water, gradually increasing natural fiber (think plants, not powders), and adding magnesium-rich foods like leafy greens and seeds can make a big difference. Go slow, though! Fiber overload can turn you into a human balloon before Pilates class. Speaking of which, movement is your best friend in supporting a sluggish system; even just a short walk outside or a quick dance around the kitchen table to your favorite songs will help your gut.

Some women also find relief with herbal allies. Senna can give a gentle nudge (used sparingly), while psyllium husks act like an intestinal broom. Slippery elm and marshmallow root help coat and soothe the gut lining, and dandelion root supports liver and bile flow to naturally stimulate digestion. Even peppermint or fennel tea can become your belly's new BFF. Just remember, "natural" doesn't always mean safe. If you're on medication, always consult a healthcare practitioner first.

Food Sensitivities: The New Plot Twist

Many women find themselves suddenly reacting to foods they've loved for years. Unlike allergies, food sensitivities tend to cause delayed, low-grade symptoms, such as bloating, brain fog, joint aches, or skin flare-ups. This makes it hard to pinpoint the culprit. This shift is often associated with alterations in gut permeability and immune function. The key? Get curious.

A simple food and symptom journal can help you uncover hidden patterns in your eating habits and health. Common triggers might include gluten, dairy, nightshades, spices, or foods that cause blood sugar spikes. Try gentle elimination and reintroduction to understand what supports you right now. And remember, eat the rainbow and combine healthy fats, protein, and nutrient-dense foods to ensure you're giving your body what it needs, especially if you (temporarily) remove any foods.

The Gut-Brain Axis: Your Inner Communication Line

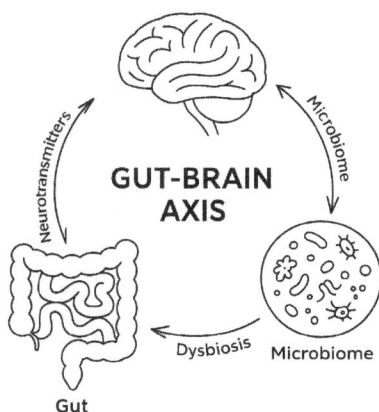

One of the most important (but often overlooked) relationships during menopause is the gut-brain axis, a strong two-way communication loop between the digestive system and the brain. This pathway uses nerves (like the vagus nerve), hormones, and immune signals to send ongoing feedback. When this connection is disrupted by hormonal fluctuations, your mood, sleep patterns, digestion, and stress levels can all be impacted.

Supporting this essential connection involves more than just taking probiotics or increasing fiber intake. It's about stabilizing your nervous system through rest, movement, and stress-reducing rituals. These habits help you better understand what your body genuinely needs rather than reacting to confusing signals. Healing your digestion during menopause requires slowing down, tuning in, and nurturing your inner ecosystem with curiosity, consistency, and compassion.

Create simple, supportive habits around mealtimes: sit down, slow down, and truly savor your food. Chew thoroughly and allow your body to shift into rest-and-digest mode so your gut can send the "I'm full" signal to your brain. When you finish eating, resist the urge to rush off or scroll your phone. Instead, give yourself a few minutes of gentle movement: try a short walk, a light stretch, or some calming mat Pilates. It may seem counterintuitive, but this small pause actually supports digestion, calms your nervous system, and helps your gut function more efficiently.

Waste Elimination

Since we have discussed bowels, let's focus on your stools. It might not be the most glamorous topic, but what happens (or doesn't happen) in the bathroom offers important clues about your health, especially during menopause. And, during midlife, it can sometimes feel downright frightening. So, if you want real insight into how your digestion, hormones, and overall well-being are doing, your daily (or not-so-daily) bathroom routine is a strong indicator.

One of the first questions I ask women who come to me with bloating, fatigue, or brain fog is, "How often are you going?" You'd be surprised by their answers. One lovely client, Robin, casually mentioned she only went every four to five days. I almost fell off my chair! No wonder she felt sluggish, bloated, and off.

Here's the deal: around once a day is ideal. Some people go more often, some less, but if your bowel movements are only every few days, your body isn't effectively clearing out waste. That's not just uncomfortable; it also impacts your hormones. Estrogen that should be eliminated through the bowels can be reabsorbed into the bloodstream, causing mood swings, bloating, or skin breakouts.

But during menopause, slower digestion is highly common. Hormonal changes, stress, reduced activity, and often not enough fiber and hydration all contribute. So, if your bathroom habits have changed, don't ignore them. It's time to support your gut!

While we're here, what it looks like matters, too. A healthy bowel movement should be well-formed, medium brown, easy to pass, and leave you feeling done. No straining, no rushing, no second-guessing. I like to say it should look like Postman Pat: smooth, sausage-shaped, and sitting proudly in the bowl. Not too hard, not too soft. Just right.

Blocked Up

If things look more like rabbit pellets, that usually indicates constipation or slow gut motility. It means your system is moving a little too slowly. This is often linked to low fiber intake, not enough fluid consumption, limited physical activity, or hormonal changes. If you're feeling bloated or like you never fully finish going, your gut is asking for support.

Gentle daily movement, warm water, hydrating foods, fiber-rich veggies, and healthy fats can help things return to a better rhythm.

Loose Bowels

On the other hand, if you're experiencing that "go now or else" urgency, your gut might be inflamed, irritated, or reacting to stress or sensitivities. This kind of reactive digestion is often linked to food triggers, gut dysbiosis (bacterial imbalance), or an overstimulated nervous system. It's also common in women with IBS or high stress levels. The key here is to calm, soothe, and rebuild. Cutting back on inflammatory triggers, such as excess dairy, gluten, alcohol, or caffeine, and introducing gut-healers like bone broth, flaxseed tea, slippery elm, and pre- and probiotics, can gently reset both your gut and your nervous system.

Supporting Gut Healing

Creating a happy gut is about consistency and care. First, you need to create the right environment for good gut bacteria to thrive by adding fiber-rich foods like garlic, leeks, bananas, and legumes, alongside hydration, low stress, and a diverse, plant-based diet to keep your gut bacteria happy and balanced. Then you can introduce a high-quality probiotic to support and maintain that healthy balance.

One daily habit I love is a high-quality probiotic with multiple strains to support digestion and a healthy vaginal microbiome. During menopause, both gut and vaginal flora can change, leading to dryness and even infections; therefore, maintaining a healthy balance of good bacteria is key. Look out for strains like Lactobacillus rhamnosus, Lactobacillus reuteri, and Bifidobacterium lactis; they are known for supporting immune function, gut barrier integrity, and urogenital health. I see probiotics as part of my self-care routine, a quiet, daily way to build internal resilience and keep things functioning smoothly on every level.

Most of all, remember this: Healing isn't doing everything perfectly. It's giving your body the right tools and the grace to find its balance. The women I've seen thrive through gut healing aren't the ones jumping from one plan to another or cutting out everything. They're the ones who take it slow, stay curious, and nourish their bodies with consistency and kindness.

If symptoms persist despite these shifts, see the appendix for deeper dives on leaky gut, SIBO, and targeted supports, and talk with your healthcare professional.

Everyday Sauerkraut

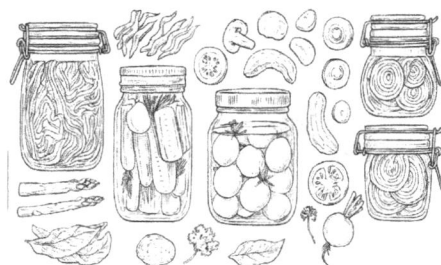

Fermented foods should become a daily staple for gut-friendly, hormone-boosting meals. Sauerkraut & Co. is excellent for your gut and, by extension, your overall health, including mood, immunity, and hormone metabolism. Fermented foods are a better alternative to taking probiotics because they are more easily absorbed and more budget-friendly.

Making your own is easier than you'd think. My go-to recipe is tangy, crunchy, and full of probiotic goodness.

You'll need:

- 1 medium green cabbage, finely shredded (about 1.2 to 1.5 kg)

- 1 to 1.5 tablespoons unrefined sea salt

- Optional: 1 teaspoon caraway seeds, juniper berries, or grated ginger for extra flavor and digestive support

Method:

- Prepare the cabbage: Remove any damaged outer leaves and set aside one clean leaf. Finely shred the rest using a sharp knife, mandoline, or food processor.

- Salt and massage: Place the cabbage in a large bowl. Add salt and massage it for five to ten minutes until it softens and begins to release liquid.

- Pack it in: Transfer the cabbage and its juices into a clean glass jar or fermenting crock, pressing down to eliminate air pockets. Leave a couple of inches at the top.

- Weigh it down: Use the reserved cabbage leaf to cover the surface, then add a fermentation weight or small clean glass to keep everything submerged.

- Ferment: Cover the jar loosely (with a cloth or a non-airtight lid) and let it ferment at room temperature, out of direct light. Start tasting after five to seven days. I usually like mine around ten days. Once it hits your perfect tang, seal and store it in the fridge.

Extra Tips:

- Always use clean hands and tools, fermentation thrives on healthy bacteria.

- A little fizz or white scum is normal, just scoop it off.

- Aim for 1 to 2 tablespoons daily with meals to support digestion.

- Try with eggs, grain bowls, salads, or just as a zingy little side. It's an easy, joyful way to sneak probiotics into your day, and a delicious act of self-care, straight from your kitchen.

Gluten and Modern Wheat

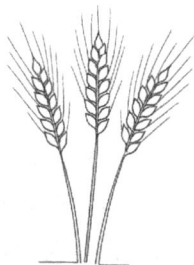

Found in wheat, barley, and rye, gluten is a protein that gives bread its chewy texture and helps dough rise. It can also be hidden in everyday foods like sauces, salad dressings, soups, gravies, soy sauce, and even oats (unless specifically labeled gluten-free, as oats are often cross-contaminated during processing).

One of the most meaningful turning points in my gut health journey came when I discovered *Wheat Belly* by Dr. William Davis. His book explains why modern wheat is different from the wheat of yesteryear: Over the past fifty years, it has been genetically modified and bred to yield more. As a result, its protein structure has changed substantially, and it now contains much more gluten. Today's wheat is a form that our bodies often neither tolerate nor digest well.

The gluten in today's wheat can trigger gut inflammation, affect blood sugar regulation, and damage the delicate lining of the intestines. It can make your gut wall more permeable, letting unwanted particles and toxins leak into your bloodstream, and fire up your immune system. When you're already dealing with fluctuating hormone levels, this often manifests as bloating, fatigue, brain fog, mood swings, cravings, and skin flare-ups.

Now, I've been tested, and according to the results, I don't have a gluten intolerance. But tell that to my belly after a bit of baguette for lunch. Within an hour, I go from feeling light and energized to walking around like someone inflated a small watermelon under my shirt. And it doesn't stop there. The next day, my energy crashes, and I feel like I'm wading through molasses. My digestion slows to a crawl and, of course, my mood takes a nosedive. My whole system just feels off. And I know I'm not alone. There's now even a term for it: to be "glutened."

Many women I coach share similar stories: no official diagnosis, no allergy. But their symptoms are clear as day. When they cut out gluten, they suddenly feel like someone has flipped the switch back on. The bloat decreases, their energy comes back, and their mood lifts. They feel like themselves again.

Here's why cutting out gluten seems to help so many women around midlife: It's partly because, as estrogen declines, our digestive efficiency naturally slows down. We tend to produce less stomach acid and fewer digestive enzymes, which makes it harder to break down certain foods, especially gluten. Add a gut that's already more sensitive due to hormonal shifts, and it's no surprise that even "healthy" wholegrain choices can start causing discomfort.

Gluten can also interfere with your gut-brain connection by disrupting neurotransmitter production, affecting focus and emotional balance in its wake. So, cutting gluten from your diet might also stabilize your mood and focus.

Happily, Gluten-Free

If you choose to go gluten-free, your life is not over, even if a few of my clients initially thought so! These days, there are plenty of delicious options available in supermarkets and restaurants if you choose to eat out. You can choose to try lowering gluten in your diet, take enzymes to help your body digest gluten, or cut it out for a while to see what happens.

You don't have to commit to a gluten-free lifestyle forever. A simple three-week experiment is often enough to discover if gluten is secretly holding you back. Just pay attention to how you feel. Word of warning: if you go cold turkey for a while and then indulge in gluten-loaded treats, you may get a bad case of feeling "glutened." This is because your gut microbiome adjusts to your diet and may be even less well-equipped to suddenly digest gluten.

If you choose to go gluten-free, life can still taste amazing. These days, many delicious gluten-free options are genuinely nourishing and satisfying. I've fallen in love with making my own gluten-free seeded sourdough. The texture is rich, yet tender. I've even cultivated a starter from rice flour to use for my favorite Seeded Multigrain Gluten-Free Sourdough Recipe from Vanilla and Bean. Baking my own bread has become one of my favorite monthly rituals. I slice it after baking, then put it straight into the freezer, so I always have gut-friendly toast ready.

When you start noticing how different foods make you feel, treats become even more satisfying because they'll no longer cost you energy or clarity. If gluten is quietly stealing your spark, maybe it's time to take a break. You can see what happens, and perhaps you'll get your glow back.

Dairy and Midlife

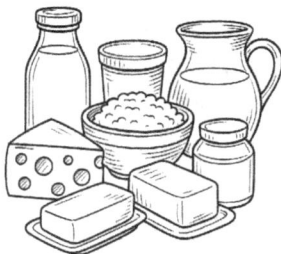

Now is a great time to reassess what you put on your plate. Dairy is often top of the list, and for good reasons. During perimenopause and menopause, when hormones, digestion, and inflammatory responses all behave unpredictably, dairy can potentially aggravate problems for two reasons: it's full of hormones, and your ability to break down lactose may have decreased.

As Dr. Neal Barnard explains in his brilliant book *Your Body in Balance*, "*Dairy products are one of the most hormone-active foods we consume. They come with hormones from pregnant cows that can interfere with our delicate hormone balance.*" Designed to help calves grow quickly, dairy products contain estrogen and progesterone, as well as so-called growth factors. Introducing this mix into a system that is already recalibrating its hormones can lead to increased bloating, breast tenderness, acne, mood swings, or stubborn midsection weight.

Then there's the lactose. As we age, we produce less lactase, the enzyme responsible for breaking down lactose. Many women find that their ability to digest dairy products has decreased. That glass of milk or scoop of ice cream that once brought joy might now leave you bloated, congested, gassy, and needing a nap after lunch. Temporary dairy intolerance can also be the result of a course of antibiotics or other factors influencing your microbiome. Some statistics indicate that up to three-quarters of the population may have some form of dairy intolerance.

But before you ditch all dairy products, be aware that there are a) differences in the way your body can break down fermented dairy products such as yogurt or some hard cheese, b) enzymes you can take to help you digest dairy products, and c) different amounts of lactose in dairy products. The worst offender is obvious: drinking milk. Soft cheeses and cream, as well as all products containing them, like ice cream, are most likely to cause digestive upsets.

Many of us are so accustomed to these symptoms that we may not even realize the constant drain on our energy. One of my clients described it perfectly: "I didn't realize how congested and inflamed I felt until I stopped dairy. And now I feel like I've taken off a heavy sweater I didn't know I was wearing, and my nose has stopped running." That sums it up beautifully. Sometimes, we don't realize how much something is weighing us down until it's gone.

And don't worry; going dairy-free doesn't mean a life of deprivation. There are now many amazing plant-based alternatives: creamy nut milks, rich coconut yogurts, dreamy cashew cheeses, and dairy-free ice creams that taste just as indulgent, minus the post-dairy slump. And when the cravings hit, have some enzymes on hand. Using them before and after foods high in dairy can address symptoms or at least reduce them significantly. This is about finding ways to feel better and live fully.

Sugar Hits at Midlife

As estrogen and progesterone levels fluctuate and decline, your body becomes more sensitive to insulin, the hormone that controls blood sugar. This means that even moderate amounts of sugar can lead to increased insulin resistance, promote fat storage (especially around the belly), cause blood sugar crashes, and lead to fatigue. Sugar also causes inflammation, which can worsen joint pain and brain fog, and increase hot flashes and night sweats. Most importantly, it raises your risk of type 2 diabetes and heart disease. A low-sugar diet must be part of any long-term health plan.

When it comes to mood and sleep, sugar can lead to a wild ride. After a quick burst of energy or comfort, the crash that follows can leave you feeling anxious, irritable, or teary, and wide awake in the early hours. It disrupts your natural rhythm, making it harder for your nervous system to find balance. Many women in midlife notice that cutting back on sugar results in more emotional stability, sharper thinking, and much deeper, more restorative sleep.

Then there's the gut and hormone connection: sugar feeds harmful bacteria and yeast, which disrupt your gut microbiome, the ecosystem that influences everything from digestion to immunity to hormone detox. A sluggish, inflamed gut makes it harder to clear excess hormones, absorb nutrients, and stay balanced. This creates a chain reaction of hormonal imbalance, bloating, cravings, and low resilience.

In short, cutting back is one of the most impactful shifts you can make. This means nourishing your body with foods that support you. Reading labels becomes an essential part of reducing sugar and reclaiming your energy. Sugar hides where you wouldn't necessarily expect, from granola to salad dressing and protein bars to gluten-free crackers. Keep an eye out for these common culprits: anything ending in -ose, containing syrup, cane juice, or natural sweeteners.

Just because something is labeled as "healthy" or "natural" doesn't mean it's low in sugar. The more you learn to spot hidden sugars, the more empowered you are to make choices that support you.

Reflect and Reset

As you close this chapter, take a quiet moment to reflect on your relationship with your gut. Your digestion depends on how you listen to and nourish your body every single day.

Start simply by noticing. Tune in to how you feel after meals: your digestion, energy, and mood. Keep a small journal if that helps. Are there foods that leave you feeling heavy, foggy, or tired? Are there meals that make you feel lighter, clearer, and more grounded? Your body constantly sends signals. The magic lies in listening.

Start with one or two gentle habits. Consider slowing down while eating, chewing more thoroughly, taking a short walk after meals, or sipping warm water throughout the day. You might consider adding a probiotic or removing a potential irritant like gluten or dairy for a few weeks to observe any changes.

And as you do, remember, healing your gut and nurturing the gut-brain connection is about building a trusting, kind relationship with your body. Because when you listen without judgment, you create space for profound, lasting change. Go gently but keep moving forward. Your gut and your future self will thank you.

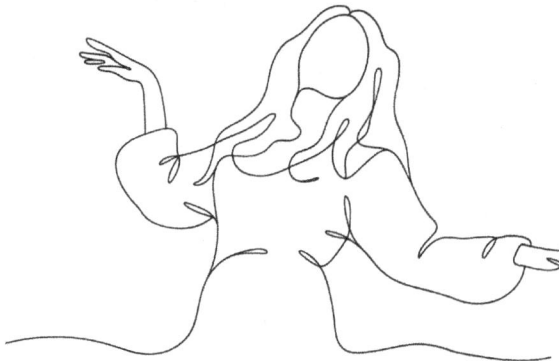

CHAPTER 9

Fuel with Protein, Fats, and Fiber

"Eating healthy food fills your body with energy and nutrients. Imagine your cells smiling back at you and saying: 'Thank you!'"

– KAREN SALMANSOHN

Macronutrients

What you eat now matters more than ever. Your midlife body requires real nourishment that supports balance and repair. It's about eating smarter, and that begins with understanding the essential building blocks that help you maintain energy, stabilize mood, support digestion, and rebuild strength. These are macronutrients: protein, carbohydrates, and fats. They're called "macro" because your body needs them in relatively large amounts, especially now, when nutrient absorption can decline and digestive shifts may affect how well you process your food. We'll talk about micronutrients like vitamins and minerals later in the book.

MACRONUTRIENTS

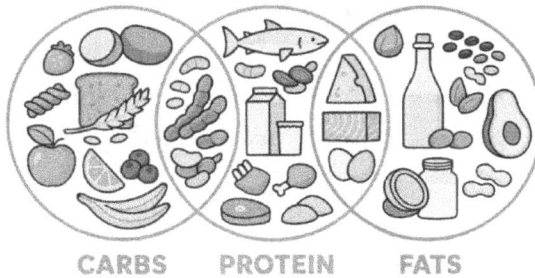

CARBS   PROTEIN   FATS

Generally, your midlife macronutrient balance means protein and carbohydrates should each form 25 to 30% of your daily food intake. Make sure you focus on **high-quality proteins**, vegetables, fruits, legumes, and gluten-free whole grains to keep things moving with a high-fiber content. The rest, roughly 20 to 30% of daily intake, should be fat from healthy sources like avocados, nuts, and olive oil. These proportions are flexible and can be adjusted depending on your needs, activity levels, or goals, whether that's weight loss, menopause symptom relief, and/or blood sugar control.

Let's dive into the power of each macronutrient. It'll help you make informed, intentional choices every time you stroll through the supermarket and fill your plate. Because how we fuel ourselves today shapes how we'll feel today, tomorrow, and even ten or twenty years down the track.

Protein Power

In nearly every tired, foggy, bloated, or not-quite-themselves client I meet, protein seems to be the missing piece. Protein helps build and maintain lean muscle, which is essential for supporting your metabolism, joint stability, and overall strength as you age. It keeps your blood sugar steady, which means fewer energy crashes, fewer cravings, and less of a mid-afternoon mood dip where everything and everyone suddenly feels overwhelming. It also plays a vital role in producing neurotransmitters, like serotonin and dopamine, your feel-good brain chemicals, making it just as important for emotional balance as it is for physical vitality.

Beyond that, protein supports bone density, especially when combined with strength training, helps repair tissues, boosts immune function, and backs up your adrenal and thyroid health. And one of its most practical perks? It enables you to feel full and satisfied so you're not prowling the pantry between meals, wondering what happened to your self-control.

Here's why so many women in midlife should be eating more protein than they do: As estrogen levels begin to drop during perimenopause, the muscle-protective magic it once offered starts to fade. We naturally begin to lose lean muscle, even if we're still moving regularly, and our metabolism starts to slow. At the same time, the body becomes less efficient at using dietary protein to build or maintain muscle. This is known as anabolic resistance.

Research indicates that women can lose up to 3 to 8% of their muscle mass per decade after the age of thirty, and this rate can accelerate to 1 to 2% per year during the menopausal transition. When I first learned this, it was a shocking revelation that motivated me to prioritize protein and make regular strength training non-negotiable to prevent my muscles from shrinking.

This means, just to maintain the same strength and vitality, we now need more protein. Research recommends eating nearly double the amount previously recommended. Eating the right amount not only supports your muscles and bones but also helps combat the natural decline in muscle mass that often occurs during midlife.

Protein Portion Size

During my burnout years, following a "low-fat, low-protein" mentality, I was doing all the supposedly "healthy" things I'd been taught, like grazing on fruit and rice crackers and loading up on vegetables. But I was hardly having any protein. At all. And I was utterly drained.

When I started studying nutrition science, I decided to weigh my protein portions. I was surprised by how much more I needed, perhaps unsurprisingly given my diet choices are at times fully vegetarian. I did this for a week and got a much clearer sense of how to build my meals with enough protein for stability and nourishment. It was such a helpful reset.

Once I began consistently eating about 25 to 30 grams of protein at every meal, my energy stabilized. I could finally build strength again. My brain fog began to lift (well, mostly), my recovery improved, my mood evened out, and I felt more like myself again. I even noticed a difference in my muscle tone.

If you've ever wondered whether you're getting enough protein, why not try tracking your intake for just a few days? It might be a real eye-opener. In general, most meals should include a palm-sized serving of protein. This is a much simpler and faster method for measuring than using scales.

Good Protein Options

Let's make protein your new best friend. With your digestion, hormones, and energy levels more sensitive than ever, choosing the right type matters. Animal-based proteins provide all essential building blocks for many of the body's processes but may not be your first choice if you are plant-based for ethical reasons. Plant-based proteins aren't complete and require a bit more mindfulness to ensure you hit your body's needs. Whether you eat animal products, lean plant-based, or mix it up, there are plenty of ways to make protein work for your lifestyle.

Animal-Based Proteins

These contain complete proteins, meaning they contain all nine essential amino acids your body can't make on its own. These amino acids serve as the raw materials for muscle repair, hormone production, immune support, and tissue healing, all essential processes that become even more crucial as we transition through perimenopause and beyond.

Animal proteins are more easily absorbed and utilized by the body, especially for rebuilding muscle and maintaining steady energy levels throughout the day. Here are some of the most beneficial animal protein sources:

- Chicken and turkey. Lean, versatile, and iron-rich. A great go-to for supporting energy and stabilizing blood sugar without added saturated fat.

- Lean red meat. A great source of highly absorbable iron and B12, both essential for women dealing with fatigue, low mood, or low blood pressure. If you only eat red meat once or twice a week, make it count. Choose grass-fed or organic options whenever possible.

- Eggs. High in protein, B vitamins, and choline (which supports brain health) and easy to digest. Most of the nutrients are in the yolk. Cook your eggs thoroughly, especially if you have an autoimmune condition. Undercooked or raw eggs carry a small risk of Salmonella.

- Fish and seafood. Especially oily fish, like salmon, sardines, and mackerel, are rich in omega-3 fatty acids to support brain, heart, and joint health. Omega-3s are also anti-inflammatory, which can help ease menopausal symptoms. Aim for at least one to two servings a week.

- Greek yogurt and cottage cheese. Great options if you tolerate dairy; high in protein and calcium. They also contain probiotics to support gut health and digestion. Try coconut yogurt with added probiotic cultures as a dairy-free alternative. Cheese, when eaten in moderation, can be a nourishing source of protein, calcium, and healthy fats, but opt for aged or less processed varieties like feta, goat, or buffalo cheese, which may be gentler on digestion for some midlife women.

- Bone broth and slow-cooked meats (with the bone in). Gentle on digestion and rich in collagen, glycine, and minerals supporting your gut, joints, and skin. Cooking meat on the bone draws out extra nutrients, including marrow, full of healthy fats, amino acids, and immune-supporting nutrients.

Plant-Based Proteins

Eating a variety of plant proteins can support hormone balance, gut health, and stable energy, while also helping reduce inflammation. While many plant proteins aren't complete on their own, combining a variety daily can provide your body with all nine essential amino acids it needs.

Plant-based protein-rich foods also offer additional benefits, such as fiber, antioxidants, and essential minerals to support digestion and blood sugar balance. Here are some of the best plant-based protein sources and recommended serving amounts:

- Lentils and chickpeas. Packed with fiber and plant protein, they support gut health and blood sugar regulation for steady energy levels. Also rich in folate, iron, and B vitamins to support energy and brain function.

- Quinoa. A rare plant-based complete protein, and a great source of magnesium, iron, and antioxidants. Gluten-free and incredibly versatile for use in bowls, salads, or as a breakfast option.

- Tofu and tempeh. Excellent sources of soy-based protein containing natural phytoestrogens. Tempeh (which is fermented) supports the gut, too.

- Nuts and seeds. Almonds, chia, flax, hemp, sunflower, and pumpkin seeds are rich in healthy fats, fiber, and protein. Sprinkle them into smoothies, on salads, or blend them into snacks. But remember, they're also high in fats and calories.

- Edamame. A complete protein and an easy go-to snack or side dish that's high in fiber and low in carbs.

Midlife tip:

If you're vegetarian or eating mostly plant-based, you'll likely need to be more intentional about hitting your protein targets. A palm-sized portion of plant-based protein often isn't enough to meet your daily needs. Tracking your intake for just a few days can highlight where you might be falling short. And remember: Variety is key. Different plants bring different amino acids, so mix it up!

Protein Powders

Pea, rice, or blended plant protein powders are a great way to top up your protein intake, especially after exercise or if you're in a rush. Choose a clean, low-sugar formula with minimal additives. Aim for one to two scoops (typically 25 to 30 grams, but check the label).

Whey Protein Powders

Dairy-based whey is a complete protein rich in essential amino acids. It's one of the most common types of protein powders, but if you're one of the many menopausal women with sensitivities or intolerances to dairy, it may not be an option. There are plant-based, gut-friendly alternatives, like pea, rice, or bean protein powders. Only use whey protein if you know your body tolerates it and opt for high-quality, low-additive versions to protect your gut. Then it's an excellent choice, especially post-workout, if you want to build or maintain lean muscle, as it supports muscle repair and recovery.

Pea, Rice, and Bean Protein Powders

These plant-based blends are fantastic for digestion, rich in amino acids, and perfect for smoothies, energy balls, or just a quick protein boost during your day. They're best for women with dairy sensitivities or those who are working to heal their gut, as they are often less inflammatory and contain fewer additives. But check the label, as hidden sugars and fillers can also be found in these.

Collagen Powders

Think of collagen as one helpful piece of the puzzle, not a magic fix. Production dips in midlife, and research shows hydrolyzed collagen can improve skin hydration, elasticity, and even joint comfort within six to twelve weeks, with some studies noting reduced wrinkle depth.

Marine collagen, sourced from fish, is highly bioavailable and especially good for skin, hair, and nails. It is my personal go-to for keeping my nails and hair strong and healthy. Bovine collagen, from grass-fed cows, contains Type I and III, strengthening bones, joints, and connective tissue, making it a reliable all-rounder. Vegan collagen boosters do not contain collagen, but use nutrients such as vitamin C, silica, and biotin to help your body make its own.

Whichever form you choose, results are best when combined with a protein-rich diet and vitamin C to support collagen formation. The reward is not just in how you look but in how supported and vibrant you feel in your own skin.

Quick Tip:

I keep some protein powder blend tucked away in the pantry, ready to mix and match depending on how I feel. It's simply perfect for post-walk smoothies or those afternoons when I need something nourishing but can't be bothered to cook a full meal (because, let's be honest, sometimes we need a break from even the healthiest habits). Or if I feel a little hungry after dinner, I'll whip up a scoop of protein powder with some almond milk. It's super quick and helps curb any late-night snack attacks.

Here is one of my favorite simple protein smoothie recipes:

Green Glow Smoothie (Midlife Mojo Edition)

Ingredients:

- 1 scoop pea- or bean-based protein powder (unsweetened vanilla is excellent)
- 1 cup unsweetened almond or coconut milk (or mix the two for creamy goodness)
- ½ a ripe banana (adds creaminess and natural sweetness)
- 1 tablespoon nut butter (almond or peanut is great for satiety and healthy fats)
- 1 teaspoon maca root powder (hormone and energy support)
- 1 teaspoon raw cacao powder (hello, antioxidants and magnesium hit)
- 1 teaspoon psyllium husk (for gut-loving fiber and blood sugar balance)

- 1 handful of spinach or kale (adds a boost of iron, calcium, and detox-loving nutrients)
- A few ice cubes or a splash of cold water (for desired consistency)

Optional add-ins:

- 1 teaspoon chia seeds or ground flaxseed
- 1-2 dates if you want it a little sweeter
- Dash of cinnamon or ginger for extra zing

How to make it:

Pop all the ingredients into a high-powered blender and mix until smooth and creamy. Serve in a fancy glass with a stainless-steel straw, and it feels like a real treat! Sip slowly and enjoy the calm energy lift and gut-soothing vibes. This smoothie keeps you nourished and grounded. It's quick, easy, and genuinely good for your hormones and energy.

Proteins to Limit

Highly Processed Meats

Salami, bacon, pork sausages, hot dogs, and deli meats are all highly processed pro-inflammatory foods and should be eaten in moderation. They can harm your gut health and worsen symptoms, as your body becomes more sensitive to inflammation and stress with changing hormone levels. These processed meats often contain preservatives and nitrates that can increase oxidative stress and inflammation, high sodium levels causing water retention, bloating, and raised blood pressure, hidden sugars and additives that raise blood sugar and disrupt digestion, and saturated and trans fats that are harder for the body to metabolize and may increase the risk of heart disease.

Low-Quality Protein Powders

These often seem like an easy health boost, but many are filled with artificial sweeteners, gums, fillers, and poor-quality dairy proteins. These mixes can cause bloating, mess with your digestion, and disrupt your blood sugar. The name and price say it all: Cheap often means low quality. Flavored or sweetened are the worst.

Read the label on your protein powders and watch out for the cheap ones full of additives and fillers, often found in cheap supermarket whey blends or identified by long ingredient lists with unrecognizable additives.

Deep-Fried Protein Sources

When protein is cooked in trans fats or highly refined oils, like in fried chicken, battered fish, crumbed meats, or deep-fried tofu or tempeh, its quality quickly declines. It also increases the strain on your liver, which is already working hard to help your body handle hormonal changes. These fatty protein sources can further raise your risk of heart disease. Additionally, fried foods can lead to weight gain, inflammation, and insulin resistance.

Highly Processed Vegetarian Proteins

Highly processed soy products, like soy burgers, soy cheese, and soy protein isolate, can affect hormone balance, especially in midlife. And while instant noodles or grain-based meat substitutes may seem convenient, they're often low in quality protein and high in refined carbs and additives, so read your labels. Choosing whole-food sources is a smarter, more nourishing option.

Putting it Together

Make intentional and conscious protein choices, as they aren't all created equal. Enjoy the less ideal ones on occasion but build your everyday protein choices around nourishing your body. Stick with grilled, baked, slow-cooked, or steamed proteins whenever you can. Your body will thank you.

Remember to spread your protein intake throughout the day. Don't save it all for dinner. Aim for roughly a palm-sized serving at breakfast, lunch, and dinner to help keep your energy consistent and your metabolism supported.

Your new motto is: "Protein equals power." You're becoming more attuned and more powerful. You're building your body's resilience. Protein supports this new version of you, the woman who knows and nourishes her body. You're becoming a powerhouse who doesn't apologize for wanting to feel strong. Now is the time to show up for yourself with presence, purpose, and yes, power. Protein helps you do just that.

Smart Snacking and Meal Plans

Let's be honest, in midlife, hunger doesn't exactly knock politely. One moment, you're fine, and the next, you're ready to rip open and wolf down a packet of pretty much anything within reach. But here's the mindset shift for you: Snacking is okay, even healthy and helpful in supporting steady levels of energy. Random, unplanned snacking is the problem. Snacking with nourishment as the aim can stabilize your blood sugar and regulate your mood. It can even prevent that dreaded afternoon crash, where you spiral into having caffeine or sugar, just to make it through the rest of the day. The key to making your snacks more nourishing is protein. I'm talking functional snacks to fuel you properly.

Here are some examples:

- Boiled eggs
- Unsweetened Greek or coconut yogurt
- Edamame
- Almond butter with apple slices or seedy crackers
- A clean, balanced protein bar
- A scoop of protein powder blended into a smoothie

The goal is to snack in a way that helps you feel better thirty minutes from now. That's the litmus test. If a snack leaves you clear-headed and energized, not jittery or crashing, go for it. If not, rethink it. This shouldn't feel restrictive in any way. It should create a sustainable rhythm. And it's not just random filler; think of it as fuel to do what you want.

Here are some one-day meal plan ideas to guide you toward simple, protein-rich choices throughout your day. I've also included a snack plan to keep your energy steady and support you between meals.

Breakfast

Scrambled eggs with greens and avocado make a hormone-friendly kickstart to your day. You'll need:

- 2 to 3 eggs (or eggs and egg whites and an added sprinkle of feta cheese for variety and taste)
- Sautéed leek, spinach, mushrooms, and zucchini in olive oil
- Quarter of an avocado sliced on top
- Sprinkle of hemp seeds for extra omega-3s
- Optional: add gluten-free seeded toast

Why it works: This combo offers protein for the brain and muscles, fats for hormonal balance, and greens for fiber and liver detox. It's the kind of breakfast that keeps you full and focused.

Mid-Morning Snack (optional if hungry)

Protein smoothie, which can also make a great on-the-go breakfast option. You'll need:

- 1 scoop collagen or plant-based protein
- Half a cup of frozen berries
- A handful of spinach
- 1 tablespoon chia or flaxseed
- 1 cup of water or almond milk
- 1 teaspoon nut butter

Why it works: This smoothie hits that mid-morning sweet spot of balancing blood sugar and boosting energy without a crash shortly after.

Lunch

Grilled chicken or salmon bowl, fueling a balanced and satisfying meal for the rest of your day. You'll need:

- Grilled chicken breast or salmon fillet
- Quinoa or brown rice (half to one cup)
- Mixed salad greens, romaine lettuce, cucumber, grated carrot, red cabbage, and spring onions
- Drizzle of tahini dressing or extra virgin olive oil and lemon

Why it works: You're getting complete protein, slow carbs, and fiber-rich vegetables with good fats for hormone and blood sugar balance. This kind of meal supports calm energy for the afternoon.

Afternoon Snack

Think protein and fiber. You could choose:

- A handful of mixed nuts with vegetable sticks
- A boiled egg and half an apple with almond butter
- A protein smoothie if you're on the go

Why it works: This is the time of day when many women hit an energy dip or start craving sugar. Make sure you have protein, as it keeps your blood sugar and energy levels stable, and your hand out of the cookie jar.

Dinner

Slow-cooked lamb, lentil stew, or oven-baked salmon with roasted vegetables provide a light, nutrient-rich meal to soothe your nervous system and support overnight restoration.

Here are some options for you:

Option 1: Slow-Cooked Lamb or Lentil Stew

- Side of roasted pumpkin, beetroot, and broccoli

- Drizzle of olive oil or a sprinkle of seeds for crunch and healthy fats

Option 2: Oven-Baked Salmon

- Served with roast sweet potatoes

- Side of fresh garden salad made from carrots, tomatoes, cucumber, red onion, and cos lettuce

- Topped with a simple tahini and olive oil dressing

Why it works: These meals are warming and grounding, making them easy to digest and giving your body what it needs to wind down without feeling overly full. You're getting a powerful combo of protein for tissue repair, fiber for digestion, healthy fats for hormone support, and magnesium-rich vegetables to calm the nervous system before bed.

Before Bed (optional if needed)

A small, nutrient-dense snack can support blood sugar stability, the nervous system, and even collagen production while you sleep. Evening snack options include any of the below (only one of them, mind you!):

- 2 tablespoons coconut yogurt with a scoop of collagen powder and a few fresh or frozen blueberries

- Half a banana with a scoop of protein powder mixed into almond butter

- 1 Medjool date with 1 tsp tahini (rich in calcium and healthy fats)

Why it works: Paired with soothing herbal tea like chamomile, lemon balm, or passionflower for extra support, this is about listening to your body and giving it a little something if it's asking. These snacks are rich in calming minerals like magnesium and potassium, support stable blood sugar through the night, and help prevent the dreaded three a.m. wakeup. The collagen gives your skin and joints a nighttime repair boost, while the natural sugars and healthy fats help signal to your body, "You're safe, nourished, and it's okay to rest."

Caring Carbohydrates

Fueling Your Energy, Mood, and Metabolism

Carbohydrates often get a bad rap, especially in diet culture, but it's time to rewrite the story. When chosen wisely, they're essential fuel. Focus on slow-burning, fiber-rich carbs to support your body, such as colorful vegetables, legumes, sweet potatoes, quinoa, and small portions of whole fruit. These complex carbohydrates help keep your blood sugar stable, your digestion regular, and your mood more even. Opting for complex carbs rich in fiber, vitamins, minerals, and slow-release energy prevents the blood sugar rollercoaster sometimes associated with carbs. Chosen well, carbohydrates can become one of your strongest allies in midlife.

Some of my go-to carbs include:

- Sweet potatoes are comforting, fiber-rich, and naturally sweet.

- Quinoa offers complete plant protein and is a fantastic grain alternative.

- Brown or wild rice is gut-friendly and sustaining.

- Steel-cut oats are perfect for breakfast with long-lasting fuel.

- Legumes, like chickpeas, lentils, and black beans, are full of protein and fiber-rich powerhouses.

- Root vegetables, like beetroot, carrots, and pumpkin, are grounding, colorful, and easy on digestion.

Here's a tip: Potatoes get a bad rap, but if you cook and cool them, some of the starch turns into resistant starch, which feeds your good gut bacteria like a prebiotic. Boil them, let them cool, then roast or reheat with olive oil. It's delicious and gut-loving!

For portion size, use a closed fist. Pair your carbs with protein and healthy fats to slow their absorption and keep your energy steady throughout the day.

Like fats, not all carbs are created equal. What you want to avoid are so-called "bad carbs," refined or ultra-processed carbohydrates stripped of their natural fiber and nutrient content. These include white bread, bagels, pastries, sugary cereals, granola bars and processed snack bars, white rice and pasta, potato chips and crackers, and baked goods such as cakes, muffins, biscuits, and croissants. Even candy, chocolate bars, and other sweet treats also qualify.

While they may have once been your go-to energy fix, your midlife body becomes more sensitive to blood sugar spikes, making these quick hits more likely to impact you negatively. These high-glycemic carbs spike insulin, stress your adrenals, and then send your blood sugar crashing, which can lead to energy dips, mood swings, increased cravings, inflammation, and even stubborn belly fat. They disrupt hormone balance and create a rollercoaster your midlife metabolism just doesn't need.

Make sure you read your labels: You'll be amazed at how much hidden sugar and processed flour is tucked into sauces, dressings, soups, and so-called "healthy" snacks. Look for ingredients like glucose, maltodextrin, corn syrup, and anything ending in -ose. Your energy and waistline will thank you.

One client, Ali, had spent years avoiding carbs and couldn't figure out why she felt moody, exhausted, and couldn't sleep. When she started adding modest portions of slow carbs to her meals, everything shifted: her energy stabilized and her sleep improved, leaving her feeling human again.

That's because carbs also play a vital role in the production of serotonin and help regulate cortisol. So, while cutting carbs might sound like a shortcut to weight loss, it can quickly backfire at midlife. The right carbs, in the right portions, at the right time, can offer steady strength and emotional grounding that lasts all day. Now, let's turn to one of the most valuable types of fiber-rich carbohydrates.

Fiber, Estrogen, and Gut Health

Most of us grow up thinking fiber helps "keep things moving," but it also plays a key role in hormone balance, gut health, and blood sugar stability—three areas often disrupted during menopause. In truth, fiber is less of a sidekick and more of a silent superhero, while also doubling as your body's internal cleanup crew. Fiber helps sweep out excess estrogen, supports the health of your gut microbiome, regulates insulin, and keeps you fuller for longer. Start by aiming for one to two cupped handfuls of fiber-rich foods per meal. That could be leafy greens, a scoop of quinoa, or a handful of berries in your morning smoothie.

There are two types of fiber, both essential for midlife health: Soluble fiber dissolves in water to form a gel-like substance. It helps slow digestion, stabilize blood sugar levels, and feeds your beneficial gut bacteria (prebiotic action). You'll find it in foods like oats, apples, chia seeds, and legumes. Insoluble fiber, on the other hand, doesn't dissolve in water. It adds bulk to your stool and supports regularity, helping to remove toxins and excess hormones from the digestive tract. It's found in vegetables, seeds, and whole grains.

These fibers work as a team to support digestion, hormonal balance, and long-term metabolic health.

Support your digestion, hormones, blood sugar, and energy levels with these simple additions:

- Ground flaxseeds are packed with both soluble and insoluble fiber, plus lignans that help bind and eliminate excess estrogen from the body. A midlife must for hormone balance and regular bowel movements.

- Leafy greens (like kale, spinach, or Swiss chard) are rich in fiber that supports healthy digestion, liver detox, and gentle daily elimination.

- Cruciferous vegetables (like broccoli, cauliflower, or Brussels sprouts) are high in fiber and glucosinolates, which help the liver metabolize hormones and clear toxins more efficiently.

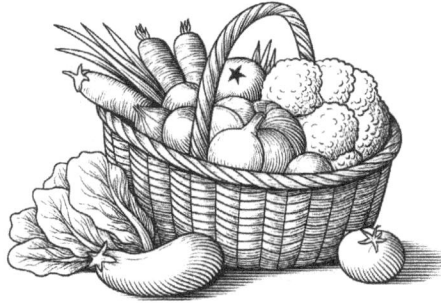

- Berries (especially raspberries and blackberries) are high in insoluble fiber that supports bowel health, feeds your gut microbes, and satisfies sweet cravings without the crash.

- Lentils, beans, and chickpeas are loaded with soluble fiber, which helps lower cholesterol, support blood sugar balance, and keep you feeling full and steady between meals.

- Whole grains (like quinoa, millet, and oats) are gentle on the gut and full of beta-glucans and resistant starches that promote a healthy microbiome and long-lasting energy.

- Psyllium husks provide soluble fiber, which forms a gel in your gut, helping to support regular bowel movements, lower cholesterol, and stabilize blood sugar. Just be sure to drink plenty of water with it.

Build your intake slowly, as too much fiber added too quickly can cause bloating and constipation. So, go gently and remember to hydrate well, too. Fiber works best in combination with water and movement to keep things flowing smoothly.

Fruit is also a good source of fiber, antioxidants, and essential vitamins. In small amounts, it can be a nourishing part of your diet. It's also high in natural sugars, which could spike blood sugar if you eat too much or forget to eat protein or fat at the same time. Hidden fruit sugar can also appear in everyday foods like smoothies. They often contain too much fruit, especially in the form of sweet, dried fruit and flavored yogurts, which can be loaded with added sugars and additives, and even 100% fruit juice, which lacks fiber to slow absorption.

When I was juicing lots, (even vegetable juices), that lack of chewing sped adsorption and slowed my digestion. Even 100% fruit juice, while natural, is stripped of the fiber that whole fruit provides. Without fiber and the act of chewing, your body absorbs the sugars more rapidly, which can spike blood sugar and leave you feeling hungrier sooner. You can get the benefits of fruit without the sugar crash by aiming for one to two servings per day and pairing fruit with a healthy fat or protein source, like nuts, seeds, coconut yogurt, or nut butter. This helps slow digestion and keeps your energy levels steady.

Eat a Rainbow of Color

Here's an easy trick that feels like a secret weapon to me: Eat the rainbow. The more color on your plate, the more you're supporting your body. Vibrant fruits and vegetables are packed with phytonutrients, the plant pigments that act like natural medicine. These compounds help reduce inflammation, protect against cellular damage, and support your liver in clearing out excess hormones.

In this rainbow of vegetables and fruit, each color plays a unique role: Reds support heart health, oranges and yellows boost immunity and brighten your skin, greens are hormone heroes, purples protect the brain, and whites are potent gut healers. Every colorful bite sends your body a message of nourishment and vitality. So next time you build a plate, aim for a rainbow. Your body will glow with gratitude.

Remember not to skimp on healthy fats and fiber either. When I started adding flaxseeds to my chia pudding, pairing berries with coconut yogurt, and piling more greens into my lunch bowl, I noticed a distinct shift. Gone were my mid-morning energy dips, my digestion improved and bloating eased, energy levels increased, skin cleared up, and I had fewer sugar cravings. These were just small, thoughtful additions, no major overhaul of my diet.

Here's why fiber is so important for your gut health: Dietary fiber acts as a prebiotic, feeding the beneficial bacteria in your gut microbiome, which in turn positively affects everything from mood and metabolism to hormone regulation. It also keeps things moving (yes, I mean digestion), supports healthy cholesterol levels, and helps stabilize blood sugar. Remember, your gut microbiome, especially the estrobolome, directly influences how estrogen is broken down. Feed them diverse fiber, and they help eliminate excess hormones, stabilize mood, and reduce hot flashes and other menopause symptoms along the way.

Here's how it can play out in practice: One of my midlife clients, Linda, felt bloated and flat, and craved sugary treats, no matter what she ate. When we simply started adding fiber-rich foods like colorful vegetables, more legumes, and a handful of seeds for most meals, things got better. Gradually, her digestion improved, her mood stabilized, and her cravings decreased. It wasn't about removing anything from her diet but adding more nourishing foods to support absorption, digestion, and the estrobolome.

How to Make it Work Daily

- Sprinkle flax, hemp, chia seeds, or psyllium husk over breakfast or salads.

- Add color to your salad, toss in a mix of vibrant veggies, such as shredded purple cabbage, cherry tomatoes, grated carrot, cucumber ribbons, fresh herbs, and a sprinkle of pomegranate seeds or sliced citrus.

- Choose roasted root vegetables, like beetroot, sweet potato or pumpkin, with dinner.

- Swap one processed snack for a handful of berries and a few walnuts.

- Sliced apple with almond butter as a snack.

These small daily swaps will gently increase your fiber intake, supporting better digestion, balanced hormones, and steady energy. I like to think of meals like art: They need a rainbow of colors, textures, and variety. You can keep it simple and flexible. But stock up your fridge and pantry with colors. Every day, aim to eat the rainbow!

Essential Fats

Fats support your brain and hormones. In this transitional phase, the right fats can be your hormones' best friend, while the wrong ones can cause serious problems. Highly processed industrial oils, such as canola, soybean, corn, sunflower, and generic vegetable oils, are everywhere. They're often hidden in packaged snacks, salad dressings, frozen meals, crackers, and even so-called "health" foods. These oils are rich in omega-6 fatty acids. Too much omega-6 can push your body into a pro-inflammatory state, raising your risk of chronic disease and hormonal imbalances. Right now, your body is already going through major hormonal shifts, so the last thing it needs is a daily dose of inflammatory fat.

Reading the back of food labels can help empower you to make better choices. You might be surprised at which foods these oils are hiding in: hummus, granola, roasted nuts, and plant-based "health" bars often sneak them in unnecessarily. If you can't pronounce the oil or if it sounds like something that belongs in a car engine, it probably doesn't belong in your body.

Instead, build your meals around anti-inflammatory fats, like extra-virgin olive oil, avocado oil, coconut oil, flaxseeds, chia seeds, nuts, and wild-caught oily fish, such as salmon. These support hormone health, nourish your brain, keep your skin supple, and help you feel full and grounded. Omega-3 fatty acids, especially EPA and DHA, found in oily fish, have been shown to reduce inflammation, support cognitive function, and modulate hormone pathways. Think of it as swapping chaos for calm; one good fat at a time.

When it comes to cooking, extra-virgin olive oil (EVOO) is a midlife must-have. It's rich in heart-healthy monounsaturated fats and loaded with antioxidants that help reduce inflammation, which is key for women during perimenopause and beyond. Unlike many processed oils, EVOO is stable at moderate cooking temperatures and supports hormone balance, brain health, and longevity (hello, Mediterranean diet!).

On the flip side, seed oils like sunflower, soybean, corn, and canola are often highly refined and stripped of nutrients. They're also high in omega-6 fatty acids, which, when out of balance with omega-3s, can promote inflammation and disrupt your hormonal harmony. Most are processed using heat and chemicals, and they sneak into many packaged foods. So, leave the seed oils on the shelf and cook with olive oil, avocado oil, or even a bit of ghee.

I also spent years avoiding fat, thinking it was the "healthy" choice. But between my memory lapses, mood swings, and thinning hair, I realized: My brain was starving. My old beliefs were based on now-updated health advice: In the 1980s, "low fat" became the standard for healthy eating. Fat was blamed for heart disease, weight gain, and high cholesterol. Supermarket shelves flooded with low-fat yogurts, margarine, snack bars, and diet foods, often packed with sugar, refined carbs, and artificial additives instead, to compensate for the missing fat.

But here's what we know now: Healthy fats are crucial for brain function, hormone production, cell repair, and sustained energy. Limiting fat too much can throw off hormone balance, increase sugar cravings, and cause nutrient deficiencies. As you can see, healthy fats are simply non-negotiable, especially in midlife when hormones fluctuate, the nervous system gets taxed, and the brain needs more support than ever.

Fats are essential building blocks for hormone production. They nourish the nervous system, support cognition, stabilize mood, keep skin supple, and help manage inflammation. And no, they won't cause weight gain if you have the portions right. The right fats can reduce cravings, keep you full, and support your metabolism. A useful guideline for including healthy fats in your diet is to aim for a thumb-sized portion or one tablespoon of fat at each meal. If you're unsure where to begin, you might try these:

- Cook your eggs in extra virgin olive oil

- Toss roasted vegetables with tahini, extra-virgin olive oil, and lemon juice dressing

- Blend flaxseed into your smoothies

- Add avocado to your lunch or a serving of salmon or sardines
- Try black cumin seed oil or evening primrose oil for extra hormonal support
- A small handful of nuts and seeds is a great snack choice (e.g., walnuts, chia, or flaxseeds).
- A spoonful of coconut oil, MCT oil, or tahini
- Some organic egg yolks

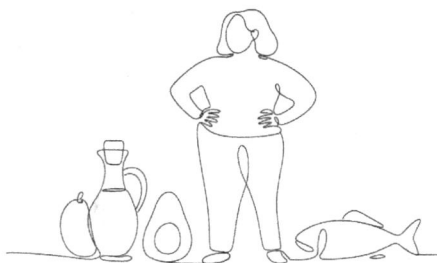

Quick Tip:

MCT oil (medium-chain triglycerides) is quickly absorbed and used for fuel, supporting brain clarity, stable energy, and fat metabolism. This is especially helpful for midlife women navigating hormone shifts, fatigue, or brain fog. Try adding one tablespoon to your morning coffee as a simple way to boost focus and fuel your day with purpose.

One client, Clare, came to me dealing with intense brain fog and unpredictable moods. Her diet was low-fat, heavy on carbs, and smoothies with very little protein. But it lacked the ingredients her body needed for satiety and nourishment. When we started reintroducing healthy fats, the transformation was quick and noticeable. She felt sharper, calmer, and more at ease in her body again.

Similarly, during my perimenopause transition, increasing omega-3 intake, especially from fish, avocados, extra-virgin olive oil, and tahini dressing and flaxseed, helped reduce hot flashes, improved sleep, and gave my skin and hair renewed vitality.

These are not minor changes by any means; they're signs your body is getting what it needs. The goal isn't to go nuts for fats, pardon the pun! It's about staying consistent. A small amount of fat with every meal goes a long way in keeping your hormones balanced, your mood stable, and your brain functioning optimally. When paired with lean proteins, fiber-rich carbs, and colorful vegetables, the right fats help turn a simple meal into a nourishing one.

Building Your Plate

You might've been reading this and still feel a bit confused about how to eat. Don't worry, because this section is all about building your plate. It's here to make food choices easy because let's face it, midlife brains can be foggy and forgetful at the best of times, and your meals should be simple, satisfying, and supportive.

Creating a balanced plate helps feed your energy, support your hormones, stabilize blood sugar, and maintain your mood. It also reduces inflammation, promotes healthy digestion, and prepares you for better sleep, sharper thinking, and greater emotional resilience.

When you skip a macronutrient, it's like pulling one leg off a stool; things become wobbly fast. You might feel fatigued, bloated, moody, or unsatisfied. But when you include all three macronutrients in the right amounts, your body feels more supported, your metabolism functions better, and your cravings decrease.

Here's how to build a hormone-supporting plate:

- Fill one-third with quality protein (think lean meats, fish, tofu, tempeh, eggs, and remember the palm-sized portion).

- Cover half your plate with colorful rainbow (or green) vegetables; the fiber, antioxidants, and nutrients help your gut and hormones.

- Add one to two tablespoons (thumb-sized) of healthy fats, like olive oil, avocado, or a handful of seeds.

- Include a fist-sized portion of complex carbs, like sweet potato, brown rice, quinoa, or legumes, for steady energy and satiety.

Meal Dream Team

Food doesn't work alone. Each macronutrient has a role, and when they work together, that's where the magic happens:

- Protein is your builder: supporting muscle, bones, immune function, and hormone production.

- Carbohydrates are your fuel: powering your brain, mood, and workouts.

- Fiber is your housekeeper: sweeping out excess estrogen and supporting digestion.

- Fats are your messengers: regulating hormones, keeping your skin and brain healthy, and helping with vitamin absorption.

- Water is your mop: flushing out toxins and hydrating every cell.

- Movement is your engine: circulating nutrients and keeping your metabolism humming.

Often, I look at my plate and ask myself, "Have I added enough color?" I pause, reassess, and add whatever I need for more variety, thinking about feeding my gut bacteria, fueling my cells, and keeping my brain sharp. I'm eating to feel vibrant and focused. When you build every plate with this intention, you're nourishing your future self. And she's strong and thriving.

Portions Made Simple

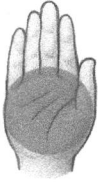

| Palm-sized for protein 3 to 4 oz | Fist-sized smart carbs 1 cup | A handful non-starchy Vegetables | Thumb-size Fats 2 Tb |

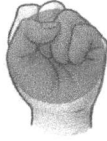

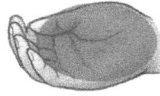

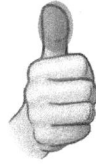

Now that we've built your hormone-supporting plate, let's discuss something that often flies under the radar: portion sizes. Over the past decade or two, our plates have gradually gotten larger and so have our servings. Without realizing it, we've been eating more simply because the plate in front of us suggested we should. Downsizing your plate can be a subtle but impactful change. No scales or calorie counting needed to get it right, just use your hand as a portion guide. For most midlife women, a balanced plate looks like:

- Palm (protein): one palm-sized serving of chicken, fish, eggs, tofu, or tempeh.

- Fist (vegetables): one closed-fist serving of non-starchy veggies (aim for two when you can).

- Cupped hand (smart carbs): one cupped-hand serving of quinoa, brown rice, beans, lentils, or sweet potato.

- Thumb (healthy fats): one thumb of olive oil, avocado, nuts, seeds, or tahini.

Adjust portions based on your hunger, activity, and goals; add a little more after heavy training, a little less when you're less active.

Full Plate to Empty Slate

Most of us in midlife are juggling more than ever: teenagers, aging parents, demanding careers, and the invisible load of holding it all together. With so much on our plates, it's no wonder meals become an afterthought. Grabbing something on the go or skipping meals entirely can seem like the only options. But those quick fixes, often loaded with processed ingredients, sugars, and empty calories, leave our bodies undernourished and overtaxed, especially during this hormonally sensitive season of life.

What we need is real nourishment. A Mediterranean-style way of eating is built around fresh vegetables, fruits, quality proteins, healthy fats, and whole grains, which offers a robust foundation for long-term health. It supports energy, mental clarity, blood sugar balance, and hormonal harmony.

I had to learn this the hard way. During my most profound fatigue in perimenopause, I wasn't fueling myself; I was just surviving. I skipped meals, grabbed snacks between meetings, and ate while scrolling or standing. I was still stuck in that old mindset of eating to shrink instead of eating to sustain. I looked lean, but I was drained. My moods were on a rollercoaster, and my digestion was in chaos. That's when it hit me: our bodies aren't asking us to be smaller. They're asking us to be stronger, more resilient, and better supported. So, I slowed down.

I stopped skipping meals. I sat down and ate properly, paying attention to what I was eating. I started focusing on the sensations of eating and chewing every mouthful, instead of unconsciously inhaling my food on the run. I filled my plate with genuine fuel: quality protein, smart carbs, healthy fats, and colorful vegetables. I remind myself (and now remind my clients constantly): take your meal breaks. Sit. Sip. Breathe. Eat to nourish, not to numb.

Now I check in before reaching for food or coffee: Am I truly hungry? Or just tired, stressed, or thirsty? Am I craving a snack, or craving space to exhale? Before grabbing the chocolate, I pause and ask: "What fuel do I need?"

It's a practice for you to embrace. Lean in and listen to your body. And here's the truth: sometimes, the answer will be food. Sometimes, it'll be water. Sometimes, it'll be rest. Whatever it is, meet yourself there with kindness. Because this isn't perfection. It's connection. It's building trust with your body, one grounded choice at a time. You deserve to eat. You deserve to feel good. You deserve time to sit, breathe, and be. That's how we go from barely making it through the day to truly living it.

Choosing Real Foods

There's an old saying: "Be kind to yourself. Your body is your temple, and you are the goddess who resides within it." Poetic? Sure. But it's also deeply true. Your body is your home. It deserves care and nourishment.

When I stopped trying to shrink myself and truly fed myself, everything changed. My energy came back. My mood stabilized. I started sleeping through the night again. That brutal chapter of crashing physically, emotionally, and hormonally forced a turning point. It gave me permission to stop ignoring my body and start listening. And so, I rebuilt.

Like many women at midlife, I had tried every restrictive diet imaginable, including smoothies, juice cleanses, and food eliminations. Nothing worked. My system was so depleted that it could barely tolerate anything. Gluten, dairy, and even healthy fats felt like too much at times. I was running on caffeine, adrenaline, and sheer determination.

At midlife, your body craves genuine nourishment. This is the time when rebuilding becomes more important than ever. As hormone levels fluctuate and your ability to recover and regenerate slows down, every cell in your body works harder behind the scenes to keep balance. That means the quality of what you eat is more crucial than ever. You're eating to restore and repair.

Real food forms your foundation. It's as close to its natural state as possible. Think colorful vegetables, leafy greens, quality proteins like free-range eggs, fish, legumes, and grass-fed meats. Include healthy fats, such as avocados, olive oil, nuts, seeds, and whole grains, that provide fiber and sustained energy. These foods are rich in the building blocks your body needs: amino acids to repair tissue, healthy fats to support hormone production, and micronutrients to reduce inflammation and protect your cells.

When shopping, walk around the edges of the supermarket, where you'll usually find fresh food, such as fruits and vegetables, followed by meat, poultry, fish, eggs, and deli items. The inner aisles tend to contain processed, packaged foods.

When purchasing anything in a packet or jar, turn it over and read the ingredients. If you can't pronounce it or don't recognize it as food, your body probably won't either. A good rule of thumb is to choose products with five ingredients or fewer and, ideally, ones you can understand.

You don't need to be perfect, but the more real food you eat (the kind of food your grandmother would recognize), the better your body will function. Midlife is the time to get back to basics: simple, nourishing, whole foods. Grown in soil, not made in a lab.

If you have access to a local farmers' market, that's even better! There, you'll often find seasonal produce, picked fresh, with fewer food miles and much more flavor. You'll also support local growers and connect more deeply with where your food comes from.

Better still, when possible, grow your own. You don't need a large garden or fancy equipment. A few pots on a balcony or porch are enough to get started. Fresh herbs, like parsley, mint, and basil, are simple, rewarding, and take up little space. Leafy greens, like spinach or arugula, grow well in containers and can be picked fresh as needed. There's something deeply satisfying about snipping herbs for dinner or picking a handful of greens you've grown yourself. You know exactly what's in your soil, and you can avoid using sprays altogether.

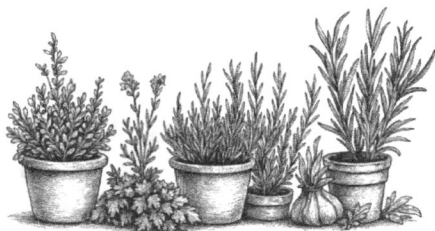

When to Choose Organic

Now, let's talk about organics. Do you need to buy everything organic? Not at all. But some produce is worth the splurge, especially when you're dealing with foods that are heavily sprayed with pesticides or grown in depleted soils. These chemicals can act as endocrine disruptors, so reducing exposure supports hormone balance and overall health. The Environmental Working Group (EWG) releases a yearly list called the Dirty Dozen. These are the fruits and vegetables most likely to retain pesticide residues, even after washing. Prioritizing organic versions of these items can help reduce your chemical load and protect your hormonal and immune systems.

The Dirty Dozen includes the following fruits and vegetables:

- Strawberries, apples, grapes, peaches, pears, nectarines, cherries, blueberries, raspberries, and blackberries.

- Spinach, kale, collard greens, mustard greens, green beans, and peppers.

These are items where the edible skin is often thin or delicate, meaning sprays are more likely to penetrate. Washing helps, but it can only do so much. For these, buying organic is worth considering.

On the flip side, the EWG also shares a Clean Fifteen list. These fresh produce items typically have minimal pesticide residues and are considered safer to buy conventionally.

It includes these fruits and vegetables:

- Avocados, pineapples, papayas, and mangoes.

- Sweet corn, frozen sweet peas, asparagus, cabbage, cauliflower, onions, broccoli, eggplant, and mushrooms.

Buying organic doesn't mean only shopping at an organic store. It means making informed choices intentionally. Maybe you choose organic berries but stick with conventional avocados. That's still a positive step. Every small decision adds up.

This year's list features many items we see on our plates every week: potatoes, berries, and leafy greens. While washing your produce with water and a little vinegar can reduce surface pesticides, remember that some residues get absorbed into the flesh. So, knowing where to spend your organic budget matters most.

At midlife, your body has enough to handle. Cutting down on toxins, even in small ways, is one of the kindest gifts you can give your future self. You don't need to completely overhaul your entire pantry overnight. Just start where you are, with awareness, curiosity, and care. Nourish yourself; don't stress. Choose real food and aim for balance.

Adding Flavor to Your Plate

When cooking, try building flavor with herbs and spices that nourish your body and delight your taste buds. Fresh herbs like basil, parsley, coriander, thyme, and dill add brightness and depth. Spices such as turmeric, cumin, smoked paprika, ginger, and garlic bring warmth and complexity to meals while also offering anti-inflammatory and gut-supporting benefits.

A squeeze of lemon, a drizzle of extra virgin olive oil, or a handful of chopped herbs can beautifully finish a dish, making your meals vibrant, light, and hormone friendly. You can also use coconut milk or coconut cream as a creamy base instead of full-fat dairy, which can sometimes disrupt hormone balance. Try to avoid rich, heavy white sauces that are harder to digest and may trigger bloating or hormonal symptoms.

I keep a drawer full of dried herbs right beside my oven, always within arm's reach, and a jar of crushed garlic and ginger in the fridge. Just half a teaspoon added to your pan or roast vegetables can be a total game changer, turning even the simplest meal into something nourishing and delicious.

Blood Sugar Timing and Fasting

Blood Sugar Balance

With the onset of menopause, maintaining stable blood sugar levels becomes one of the most overlooked yet powerful tools for managing energy, mood, and weight. As estrogen levels decline, our insulin sensitivity also drops. This makes it harder for our cells to absorb glucose efficiently, leading to higher blood sugar spikes followed by dramatic crashes. When that crash hits, your body releases cortisol to raise blood sugar again, a hormone that, in high doses, promotes fat storage, especially around the belly. You see, resisting sugary snacks isn't about willpower at all, but hormones.

This rollercoaster of insulin and cortisol explains why many midlife women experience stubborn weight gain, even if their eating habits haven't changed. Where your younger self might have bounced back from toast for breakfast or pasta for lunch, those same meals can now leave you bloated, tired, and hungrier later.

Here's how to work with your body instead of against it: Build every meal around the three stabilizers: protein, healthy fats, and fiber. This combination helps keep your blood sugar levels steady, avoiding spikes or crashes, so cortisol isn't unnecessarily triggered, and your body can finally relax its "store fat" survival mode.

Here's how it looks in practice:

- Trade fruit-only breakfasts for eggs with avocado or chia pudding with protein.

- Swap processed snacks for a boiled egg, a handful of nuts, or veggie sticks with hummus.

- Add quinoa, roasted veg, and salmon or tofu to your dinner instead of defaulting to white rice and a side of stress.

The goal is to give you greater stability. When blood sugar stabilizes, weight becomes easier to manage because your metabolism and hormones can finally get back into sync.

Meal Timing

Let's not forget the timing of your meals. Eating within an hour of waking helps reduce those early-morning cortisol spikes and sets your metabolism up for a more balanced day. From there, finding a steady rhythm by, say, eating every 3 to 4 hours (or 2 to 3 hours if you're managing fatigue), can help keep your blood sugar stable, your energy up, and your mood even. When you feed your body regularly, it learns to trust you again. It doesn't need to hold onto weight, panic, or crash at 3 p.m. Instead, you feel grounded, clear, and well-fueled.

Here's another tip: Even something as gentle as a 10-minute walk after meals helps move glucose into your muscles, reducing post-meal spikes and keeping energy stable. It's moving to improve how your body uses fuel.

Now, a quick note on intermittent fasting: Yes, it has benefits. But if you're going through menopause, feeling exhausted, foggy, struggling to sleep, or managing weight, fasting might add more stress. Your body is already under pressure. We'll explore intermittent fasting in more detail in the next chapter.

First, focus on stabilizing, nourishing, and rebuilding. Then, when you're strong and steady, you can consider other tools like fasting from a position of strength.

Nourish Without Fuss

Midlife meals don't need to be complicated. We're busy women, not contestants on a cooking show. I often eat the same meals two or three times a week, and I love making extra so I have a nourishing meal ready in the fridge the next day. Repeating meals is a smart and sanity-saving hack in my book.

Check out my seven-day plan. It's high in protein, full of color, gluten-free, dairy-free, and rich in fiber. It'll keep your blood sugar stable, meaning your mood and energy levels will stay lifted. You can mix and match, double up, or batch-cook—whatever makes your life the easiest.

Seven-Day Meal Plan

Day 1

Breakfast: Vegetable-loaded omelet with spinach, capsicum, and zucchini + half an avocado

Lunch: Quinoa and grilled chicken salad with a rainbow of vegetables (beetroot, arugula, carrot, cucumber), drizzled in lemon tahini dressing

Dinner: Baked salmon with roasted pumpkin, broccoli, and green beans

Snacks: Apple slices with almond butter and a protein shake

Tip: *Cook extra salmon tonight so tomorrow's lunch is sorted with zero fuss.*

Day 2

Breakfast: Chia pudding made with almond milk, coconut yogurt, berries, ground flaxseeds, vanilla essence, and a sprinkle of cinnamon. Add one scoop of plant-based protein powder.

Lunch: Leftover salmon tossed through a green salad with avocado, cucumber, tomatoes, red onion, and a sprinkle of seeds and chopped almonds, with tahini and olive oil dressing

Dinner: Turkey mince lettuce cups with grated carrot, zucchini, and capsicum, with cauliflower rice and a drizzle of olive oil

Snacks: A handful of walnuts and two kiwifruits, or some carrot sticks with tahini

Tip: *Double the turkey mince, freeze half for a quick dinner another week.*

Day 3

Breakfast: Protein smoothie with pea protein powder, frozen banana, spinach, nut butter, cacao, psyllium husk, and almond milk

Lunch: Lentil and quinoa bowl with roasted colorful mixed vegetable bowl with olive oil and lemon

Dinner: Grilled chicken thighs with mashed sweet potato made with olive oil and butter, sautéed kale, and garlic

Snacks: Boiled egg and cucumber sticks, or a slice of seeded gluten-free toast and almond butter

Tip: *Roast extra vegetables at lunch to use cold in wraps or salads tomorrow.*

Day 4

Breakfast: Scrambled tofu with turmeric, onion, cherry tomatoes, spinach, and a slice of seeded gluten-free sourdough

Lunch: Tuna, sweet potato, and chickpea salad with red onion, parsley, olive oil, lemon, and arugula

Dinner: Lamb kofta with roast carrots, zucchini, and a tahini drizzle

Snacks: A pear and ten almonds or a hard-boiled egg and a piece of fruit

Tip: *Make an extra kofta or two, perfect protein snack for tomorrow's lunchbox.*

Day 5

Breakfast: Overnight oats made with gluten-free oats, chia seeds, coconut yogurt, grated apple, and cinnamon (add one scoop of plant-based protein powder)

Lunch: Chicken and vegetable soup with a side of seeded crackers or seeded gluten-free toast and avocado

Dinner: Stir-fried prawns with snow peas, capsicum, bok choy, and brown rice with tahini dressing

Snacks: Celery sticks with sunflower seed butter or a protein-packed smoothie

Tip: *Freeze leftover soup in single portions for quick "emergency" meals.*

Day 6

Breakfast: Smoothie bowl with protein powder, chia seeds, rolled oats, frozen blueberries, flaxseed, greens powder, and almond milk, topped with coconut flakes

Lunch: Warm colorful mixed roasted vegetables and quinoa bowl with pumpkin seeds and grilled tofu

Dinner: Baked barramundi with roast beetroot, asparagus, and herbed green beans

Snacks: Rice cake with avocado and hemp seeds, or boiled egg and a piece of fruit.

Tip: *Bake extra barramundi and toss through tomorrow's lunch salad for variety.*

Day 7

Breakfast: Savory breakfast bowl of boiled eggs, roasted sweet potato cubes, sautéed spinach, sauerkraut, and avocado

Lunch: Turkey and avocado lettuce wrap or gluten-free wrap with shredded cabbage and grated carrot

Dinner: Slow-cooked beef on the bone stew with carrots, celery, and pumpkin over cauliflower and green pea mash, made with coconut oil

Snacks: A handful of blueberries, a Brazil nut or two, or a protein powder smoothie

Tip: *Make double stew and freeze half; you'll thank yourself on a busy weeknight.*

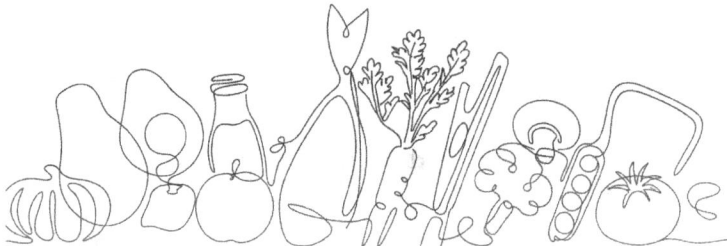

CHAPTER 10

Food Rebalance, Weight Loss, and Intermittent Fasting

"We struggle with eating healthily, obesity, and access to good nutrition for everyone. But we have a great opportunity to get on the right side of this battle by beginning to think differently about the way that we eat and the way that we approach food."

– MARCUS SAMUELSSON.

At midlife, this reminder really hits home. Food not only satisfies hunger or stress; it sustains your body. Every bite is either a little withdrawal from your energy account or a deposit that helps you feel stronger, clearer, and more balanced. Think of it like choosing between a green protein smoothie and a doughnut as your "interest rate." One pays you back, the other leaves you broke by 3 p.m.

That's where things like mindful meals and intermittent fasting aren't punishments but tools to help your food work for you, not against you. And don't worry, this isn't about eating kale forever; there's room in the budget for chocolate, too.

Let's talk about weight. Without guilt. Zero pressure. Just real talk about what's happening at midlife and what you can do to feel strong and healthy in the long run. Remember, some of the hormonal changes can put pressure on your body and increase your risk of developing disease. Being at a healthy weight, neither too low nor too high, can help lower your risk of a few of these. But before you skip ahead to the next chapter, remember that keeping your weight stable and within a healthy range is far better than yo-yoing. So, this chapter is here to support you in your choices and empower you to develop sustainable habits to rebalance your weight and, if that's the path you choose, lose weight.

Hormones at Play

If it feels like your body is playing by new rules at midlife, hormones are a big part of the story. Lower estrogen makes it easier to store fat around the belly and can interfere with how well your fullness signals work. Progesterone dips leave your body more sensitive to stress, often nudging cortisol higher, which is linked to cravings and stubborn belly fat. Testosterone naturally declines, too, which means less muscle mass and a slower metabolism. And cortisol itself, often called the "stress hormone," tends to spike more easily now, encouraging your body to hang on to fat stores while driving cravings for quick-energy foods, like sugar and refined carbs.

These hormonal shifts set the stage for how your body stores and uses energy. But they're not the only players. Your appetite is also guided by hunger hormones, the chemical messengers that tell your brain when it's time to eat and when you've had enough.

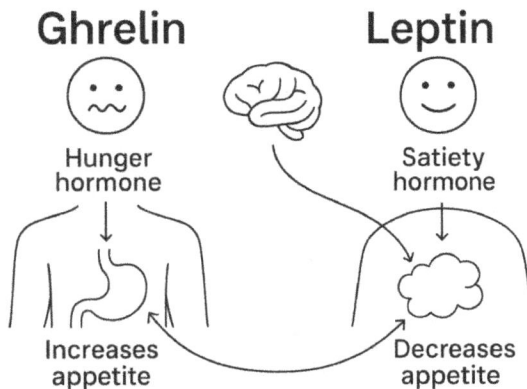

Ghrelin

Hunger hormone

Increases appetite

Leptin

Satiety hormone

Decreases appetite

- Ghrelin: The Hunger Hormone. Think of ghrelin as your body's dinner bell. It is made in your stomach and rises before meals to nudge you, "Time to eat!" Once you've eaten, ghrelin levels drop again.

- Leptin: The Fullness Hormone. Leptin is your body's satisfied sigh. It is produced by fat cells and tells your brain when you've had enough fuel stored. When leptin signals are clear, you naturally stop eating because you feel content. It's like a gentle whisper to your brain, "I'm full, you can relax."

Here's the catch: These signals aren't instant. They need about 15 to 20 minutes to do their job. That's why slowing down at meals, chewing, tasting, and savoring gives your hormones a chance to catch up and helps you feel satisfied without overeating.

Put these changes together, and it's no wonder your body feels like it's rewriting the rulebook. But knowing this isn't a reason for frustration; it's a reminder that weight at midlife is about biology, not failure. Simple lifestyle shifts like strength training, nourishing food, stress care, and better sleep can help bring these hormones, both the big-picture ones and the hunger signals, back into balance. Still, understanding your hormones is only part of the story. The other piece is how our modern food habits either nourish those systems or leave them struggling.

Global Food Habits

Today, grabbing convenience food has become the norm. Fast food chains like McDonald's are popping up like mushrooms. It's no surprise that fried snacks, burgers, and chips have become go-to choices for many of us when life gets busy. While these foods might be quick and satisfying in the moment, they're often packed with hidden calories and offer little nutritional value. Worse yet, many convenient foods are highly processed and high in saturated and trans fats, which are linked to inflammation, weight gain, heart disease, and other long-term health issues.

The global impact of this shift in eating patterns is staggering. Obesity has become a worldwide epidemic. More than a billion people are now living with obesity. In fact, adult obesity has more than doubled since 1990, and adolescent obesity has quadrupled. Women in midlife are particularly affected, as hormonal shifts, stress, sleep disruptions, and decreased muscle mass begin to influence metabolism and fat storage.

On the flip side, many women are on the other end of the spectrum, who have kept their bodies lithe yet likely deprived of essential nutrients, and they also risk long-term disease. Osteoporosis and other health risks fall like dominoes once you start having recurring fractures. You can't really win at either end of the spectrum. It's not surprising a lot of us resign ourselves to drowning our physical symptoms and keep making the same old choices (maybe not even expecting a different result).

Let's be honest, though, eating on the run doesn't set us up to feel our best. At best, convenient foods give us a full (read: bloated) tummy and quick energy before the inevitable crash and worsened menopause symptoms. It's running our bodies on bad fuel and continuing on fumes before the next pit stop. Eating this way, we're ignoring that our bodies are truly craving slow, real food: fresh vegetables, whole ingredients, meals cooked with love, and shared moments around the table.

I'm not here to wag my finger. I get it. Convenience is king. Food is often an afterthought. But what if you could take just one little step at each meal to support and nourish your body better? Set aside the worries of long-term disease and concerns about fitting into your clothes (negative motivation never works in the long run) and think about how you'd like to feel now. Would you make more nourishing choices if you paused, tuned in briefly, and remembered why you're eating?

Nourishment. We're here to nourish you for a joyful life, one where you no longer need to ride waves of sugar highs and symptom lows but can move along steadily, with clarity and much more ease than before. Perhaps feeling better and more in control than ever before. Certainly, more empowered.

If you haven't already, I highly recommend watching the Netflix documentary *Live to 100: Secrets of the Blue Zones*. It's a fascinating look at how people in certain parts of the world live longer, healthier lives, often reaching one hundred and beyond, with vitality and joy. What stands out most is that their health is rooted in a naturally supportive lifestyle. They eat mostly plant-based foods in modest portions, move consistently throughout the day, whether walking, gardening, or simply staying active, and make meals a shared, unrushed experience. Food is savored, not inhaled between tasks. Their environments help them thrive, with walkable streets, strong social bonds, and easy access to fresh, local produce. It's a beautiful reminder that wellness doesn't have to be complicated; it just needs to be intentional and consistent.

In midlife, this message is especially timely. According to the Centers for Disease Control and Prevention (CDC), women aged 40 to 59 have the highest obesity rates compared to other age groups. Weight gain and changes in body composition are common for menopausal women. Regardless of what you think about your appearance, these changes are tied to a higher risk of cardiovascular disease, insulin resistance, and joint strain.

Supporting your body is about understanding where your healthy weight sits now and creating new eating habits to carry you through your second act. It's about tuning in, listening to what your body needs, and boosting your health with foods that strengthen you. When you nourish yourself with intention and care, you'll feel more stable and vibrant now, tomorrow, and in the years ahead.

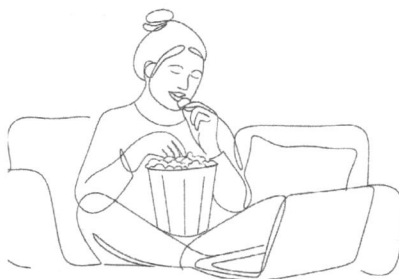

Boxed In, Slower, and Stiffer

Let's also take a moment to examine how our movement patterns have changed over the past century. We've gone from walking, farming, moving all day, even gathering food, to working and mostly socializing indoors and around "boxes." We drive to work in our cars, sit at desks all day, and stare at another box—our computers—often for hours. We eat lunch in front of screens while juggling another small box—our phones. Then we drive home to yet another box by settling in front of the TV, often with dinner in hand, watching Netflix for hours on end.

This modern lifestyle, while convenient, has made us more sedentary than ever, reducing our energy needs and harming our overall health. If you've been living this way for 20 or 30 years (as many of us have by midlife), it's no surprise that our bodies start to reflect it. Less daily movement means slower metabolism, less muscle mass, and greater difficulty regulating weight, even if our food intake hasn't changed much.

When we talk about weight loss or balance in midlife, we can't ignore this shift. Our bodies are built for natural, consistent movement throughout the day. Reintroducing intentional activity can have a significant impact. This could mean taking the stairs instead of the elevator, walking or biking to work, enjoying a brisk ten-minute walk during lunch, or just standing and stretching every hour. Even small adjustments like walking after meals, doing light housework, or parking a little farther away can gradually retrain your body to move more and sit less.

Retraining yourself to nourish through better food and movement choices is about awareness. Our environment and habits have slowly shaped us into more sedentary beings, but the good news is, we can morph right back. One step, one stretch, one small change at a time.

Exercise is one of the most powerful tools we have for how we feel and function. During menopause and beyond, movement becomes medicine. Regular physical activity helps create a healthy calorie deficit, supports lean muscle (which burns more energy even at rest), and boosts our metabolic rate. If you're on the underweight side, weight-bearing exercise and regular movement can help boost your health and also your appetite for healthy, nourishing foods.

Strength training is especially key at midlife; it helps combat age-related muscle decline, supports insulin sensitivity, and protects bone health. Building more muscle also boosts your metabolism, since muscle tissue burns more calories even at rest. In other words, the stronger your muscles, the more freely your body can use food as fuel.

But it's not all about lifting heavy. Cardiovascular movement improves heart health and helps burn calories, while Pilates, yoga, and balance-focused exercise enhance flexibility, posture, and mental clarity. Even short, consistent sessions can make a big difference. Whether it's a morning walk or a few sets of strength training, your body will thank you. Movement lifts your mood, reduces stress, supports better sleep, and reminds you that you're still strong and vibrant. This is about moving with purpose and care.

Remember to start small. If exercise hasn't been part of your routine for a while (or ever), don't panic. You don't have to join a bootcamp or become a Lycra-clad gym goddess overnight. Start where you are. That could be a gentle 10-minute walk around the block, some stretches while the kettle boils, or light movement during TV ad breaks (yes, you can become a commercial break athlete). Before you start anything new, especially if you have existing health conditions, check in with your health care provider to ensure you're good to go. They'll likely be thrilled you're taking a proactive step.

Learning from International Eating Habits

Nourishing your body is also about how you eat. When you look around the world, you'll notice something fascinating: cultural food habits deeply shape body size and health. Every country has its version of dietary guidelines, often shown as food pyramids or plates, based on local food availability and cultural traditions. They provide a snapshot of a culture's balanced way of eating. But they also remind us that health isn't a one-size-fits-all formula. It's shaped by our daily rhythms and community's habits.

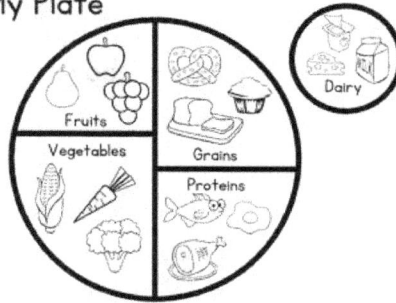
My Plate

In 2011, the USDA replaced their former classic food pyramid with MyPlate, a simple image of a plate divided into four sections, with a side of dairy. The idea is straightforward: Fill half your plate with vegetables and some fruit and divide the other half between protein and whole grains. It's a visual guide to make meals healthier and more balanced.

France is one of my favorite places in the world, especially the villages where traditional food culture still thrives. Meals are shared slowly, each bite savored. Plates are a modest size, snacks are rare, and a trip to the local produce market often means walking or biking. Wine is sipped, not chugged. And eating emotionally or while multitasking isn't part of the cultural norm.

Unfortunately, many of these traditional ways of eating are becoming outdated with globalization. But, while we often search for the next diet hack or boot camp, we can learn much from traditional ways of eating.

Our developed habits of eating on the run, treating meals as purely functional, and portion sizes so big we need an antacid to finish us off, all point to a lack of connection to our body and our emotional needs. Our environment encourages this disconnected, overloaded way of eating.

We often encounter buffet-style eating, where plates are piled higher than our stomachs can handle. Then we go back for seconds, not because we're hungry, but because there's too much choice and not enough self-regulation. Fun fact: It takes about twenty minutes for your stomach to send a "full" signal to your brain. If you eat too fast, your "I'm full" hormone leptin doesn't have time to do its job, and you may overeat before your brain catches up. Try slowing down, chewing mindfully, and giving yourself a good twenty minutes to eat. Your digestion and your waistline will thank you.

Eating whole foods slowly, intentionally, and stopping when you're comfortably full are the true "secrets" to sustainable weight balance. They create a more peaceful relationship with food. As you continue making empowered food choices, take inspiration from cultures that eat with presence and connection. Your midlife body needs more than nutrients. Nourish it with connection, take pleasure in your food, and eat with great care. Bon appétit!

Caloric Balance

By the time you hit midlife, chances are you have tried a diet or two (or perhaps countless ones), struggled with weight gain or loss and experienced a yo-yo effect. There's evidence that most bodies have a set point they try to reach; if you push them one way or the other, especially if you do so by restricting what you eat. Our tendency to store fat is also determined to a large degree by genetics, early childhood nurture, hormones, and habits. It sounds like an insurmountable mountain, as those of us who have tried pushing our set point up or down know well. This doesn't mean we are stuck at the weight we are at.

This is an important and empowering point to understand, as weight is a factor linked to long-term disease. While your body has a natural tendency to work toward a set point, it's not necessarily fixed. Research suggests you might be able to gradually reset your set point by slowly losing weight through sustainable healthy lifestyle changes, avoiding quick fixes, and building muscle mass through strength training. Aim to follow the 80/20 approach: about 80% of your meals are nourishing whole foods, and 20% leave room for treats you love. This balance is especially helpful in midlife because it supports steady weight loss without the guilt or burnout that strict dieting can create.

So, let's talk calories, because it's incredibly helpful to understand how weight loss and gain work. To estimate your daily calorie needs, you first need to calculate how many calories you burn at rest, your Basal Metabolic Rate (BMR). Then you adjust the result for your activity level. You can use this formula: $(10 \times$ your weight in kg$) + (6.25 \times$ your height in cm$) - (5 \times$ your age in years$) - 161$. Multiply your BMR by your general activity factor: 1.2 for sedentary, 1.55 for moderately active, or 1.9 for very active. Voilà: that's your Total Daily Energy Expenditure (TDEE). You'll get a rough daily calorie need baseline this way.

But, of course, our actual needs vary. Some of us have faster metabolisms, others are more active. Sometimes, we have injuries reducing movement, and as we age, our baseline naturally drops. That means we may not need as many calories as we once did. Eat a little more than you need on most days, ideally through nutrient-dense foods, such as nuts, and your weight should creep up over time. That's if you don't have any underlying conditions. Reduce your intake just slightly (for example: replacing high-calorie choices with extra vegetables instead), eat a little more slowly so you stop when you're satisfied, or move a little more to increase your output, and you should gradually lose a bit of weight (or increase your muscle mass).

But remember, quality matters just as much as quantity. You still want to focus on nutrient-dense meals rich in protein, fiber, and healthy fats to keep hormones and energy stable. Your body won't respond well to deprivation or sudden weight loss. Changing your diet should focus on making positive changes for your body and mind.

One of my clients, Susan, realized she was often mistaking thirst for hunger. Once she focused on staying hydrated, along with a balanced, healthy diet and regular movement, the weight started to shift. Over a year, with weekly check-ins, she lost 55 pounds, her diabetes improved, and her overall health markers got better; no crash diets, just steady, sustainable change.

The key is to aim for slow, sustainable weight loss, not drastic, quick fixes. That way, you build eating and lifestyle habits that are sustainable in the long run. It's also best to get personal guidance. A nutritionist or health professional can help you tailor your "weight management plan" based on your lifestyle, goals, and metabolism. Understand and nourish your body, and make empowered, long-term choices that stick.

Beyond the Scales

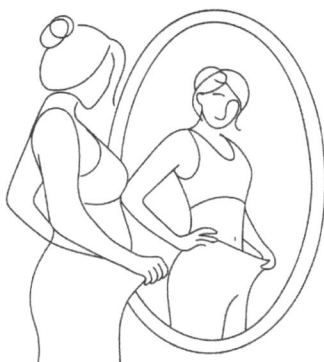

There are many different ways to measure weight, and it's not all about the scales. At midlife, hormonal shifts can cause fluctuations in water retention, digestion, and sleep, all of which can make the number on the scale feel confusing or inconsistent. That's why other indicators of progress can be just as valuable, if not more so.

Some of the most helpful tools include taking body measurements (like waist, hips, and thighs), tracking how your clothes are fitting, or snapping progress photos from the front, back, and side in consistent clothing. Whether you're aiming to lose or gain weight, measuring improvement in strength and stamina are better indicators of personal fitness and long-term health. In fact, grip strength is most closely related, so why not check this out under the guidance of a health professional? These key markers often tell a clearer story than the scales ever could.

There are also other useful tools, like a body composition scale, which gives a deeper view of what's going on in your body. Unlike a standard scale that only shows total weight, a body composition scale can estimate your body fat percentage, muscle mass, protein mass, and metabolic rate. Over time, this helps you track the effects of your fitness and nutrition habits with far more insight. It's especially useful in midlife, when the scale might stay the same, but you're gaining muscle, improving metabolism, or reducing visceral fat, changes that matter far more for long-term health than the number alone. If you're new to strength training, you should know muscle weighs more than fat, so as your body changes shape, the scales might stay the same.

There's also growing interest in weight loss medications, which some health care providers now include in broader treatment plans. These medications may help by reducing appetite, increasing calorie burn at rest, or limiting fat absorption (like Orlistat/Xenical). They can be useful tools, as mentioned, they're designed to complement healthy lifestyle changes like balanced meals and regular movement.

If you're considering medication, it's essential to have an open conversation with your doctor about benefits, risks, side effects, and cost. So far, research shows that surgical interventions, such as gastric bypass and banding, can have higher and more significant long-term success rates than weight loss drugs. However, my anecdotal experience shows that some of my clients suffer from not being able to get enough nutrients due to the portions they can eat after surgeries like this. The most effective approach is personalized and best discussed with your health care professional. What works best will depend on your body, health history, and goals.

And remember, weight naturally fluctuates during perimenopause and menopause. Hormones, sleep, stress, and inflammation all play a role. Try not to measure daily, once a week is more than enough to stay in tune without tipping into obsession. This is about honoring your body, not battling it. If you're looking for extra accountability, work with a wellness coach or qualified nutritionist. They can personalize a plan to suit your individual needs, help you build a healthier relationship with food (if that's where the work is needed), and support you with regular check-ins to keep you on track. Sometimes, just knowing someone is in your corner makes all the difference.

Alternatively, there are many supportive weight loss and wellness programs available around the world. Some, like Noom, focus on reshaping your habits and mindset around food using daily lessons and psychology-based coaching. Others, like Jenny Craig or Nutrisystem, offer more structured approaches with pre-packaged meals and one-on-one guidance.

Whatever approach you choose, the key is finding something that fits you. Support groups can also be incredibly helpful, whether in person or online. Weekly check-ins and a sense of community can go a long way in keeping you motivated. Sometimes, just knowing someone will ask how your week went is the gentle nudge you need to stay on course.

Fitness Apps

Fitness and nutrition apps can be powerful tools for building awareness. They help track what you're eating and drinking, offering insights into calories, macronutrients (like proteins, carbs, and fats), and even micronutrients (vitamins and minerals). This kind of knowledge can be incredibly useful, whether you're aiming to create balanced meals, support specific health goals, or simply build better eating habits.

I often recommend apps like Cronometer or MyFitnessPal to clients as a short-term tool. Many use them for just a few weeks to see the bigger picture of their eating patterns. I've done it, too, and was surprised to find I wasn't eating enough on some days to fuel my energy and recovery. It was a great reminder that tracking isn't just about cutting back; it's about learning what your body needs. Whether you're under- or over-fueling, or just curious, these apps can help you spot gaps and guide smarter choices.

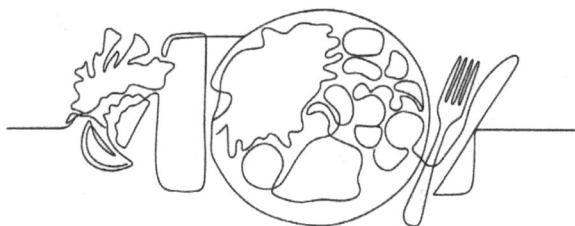

Tips for Sustainable Weight Loss

Eat with Intention

- Use smaller plates and eat slowly, giving your body time to feel full.

- Sit down to eat without distractions like TV, emails, or doomscrolling. Taste, savor your food, and chew mindfully.

- Build balanced meals. Half a plate of colorful vegetables, a palm-sized portion of protein, a fist-sized portion of smart carbohydrates, plenty of greens and colorful vegetables, and a thumb-sized portion of fat.

- Slow down and give yourself around 20 minutes to enjoy your meal, giving your hunger hormones time to signal to your body that it's full.

- Stay hydrated between meals. Thirst often masquerades as hunger, and sipping water away from mealtimes also makes digestion easier. Think of it as letting your gut focus on the main act, your food, without having to juggle a swimming pool at the same time.

- Skip drinking your calories. Sugary drinks and milky coffees add up fast without truly nourishing you.

- Keep processed foods, sugar, and alcohol to a minimum.

Move Naturally and Often

- Aim to walk more, stretch, do light housework, or take the stairs.

- Add strength training 2 to 3 times a week; it's a midlife metabolism booster.

- Try a mix of cardio and resistance training to keep your body working well.

- Park farther away and walk to your destination. Walk after meals. Little things do add up.

Create a Supportive Environment

- Clear your pantry and fridge of anything that doesn't support your goals.

- Batch cook once a week to have healthy meals and snacks on hand.

- Keep nourishing snacks and ingredients within easy reach.

- Tell friends and family you're prioritizing your health, and ask for support.

- Brush your teeth after dinner to signal "I'm done eating."

Make It Sustainable

- Avoid extreme detoxes or long fasting periods of more than 16 hours.

- Aim for a 12-hour overnight fast to let your body rest and reset.

- Use tracking apps if it helps you build knowledge and awareness.

- Set realistic goals. Know your why: Is it energy, confidence, or health?

- Ditch the scales if they cause stress. Focus on progress you can feel, how your clothes fit, your energy levels, and grip strength tests.

Just start gently, consistently, and with kindness. This is about strengthening your habits and building a way of living that helps you feel vibrant for years to come.

Smart Eating Out Tips

Remember, it's absolutely okay to enjoy a treat now and then. If you're eating well about 80% of the time, choosing balanced, nourishing meals and moving your body in ways that feel good, then the other 20% can leave space for treats or eating out without guilt. Balance really is the key. And if you want to eat out and still keep things healthy, a little planning goes a long way. Checking the restaurant's menu online beforehand helps you make simple, smarter choices.

Skip the deep-fried dishes, heavy cream sauces, and oversized pasta plates. Instead, go for grilled fish, chicken, or beef with a side of vegetables. Swap fried chips for baked potato or sweet potato, and try not to fill up on the bread basket that usually lands on the table before your meal.

If you know there's going to be a long wait before eating, have a small, protein-rich snack beforehand so you can enjoy your dinner without feeling ravenous.

When it comes to sauces and dressings, ask for them on the side so you can decide how much you want to use. Pay attention to drinks, too; alcohol, cocktails, and sugary sodas can sneak in extra calories and disrupt your sleep, so sparkling water with lemon or lime can be a refreshing alternative.

Remember that restaurant portions are often much bigger than what you'd serve yourself at home. Consider sharing a dish, asking for a half portion, or boxing up leftovers straight away. If dessert is calling your name, share one with a friend or choose a lighter option, like fruit.

And above all, slow down, savor your food, and listen to when your body says "enough." Eating out is meant to be enjoyed, balance means making choices that leave you satisfied, not stuffed.

Reclaiming Your Energy

Take a deep breath and give yourself a quiet moment to reflect on what stood out to you in this chapter. What felt true for you? Which strategies or ideas felt the most doable or inspiring for your lifestyle right now? Maybe it's starting your day with protein. Maybe it's more water. Or maybe it's becoming more aware of how meals affect your mood and energy levels. You could try keeping a food and energy journal. Just a few notes each day to track how you feel. Over time, this awareness will become your compass. It helps you make choices that serve and support your changing body.

Remember, you're not walking this path alone. Every woman's menopause journey is different, but the foundations we've explored here create a strong framework for rebuilding your energy. Small, steady changes are the quiet heroes of transformation. So, trust the process and be kind to yourself. Every so often, celebrate your progress, no matter how small it is, in making mindful choices along the way. Once you've laid those foundations, you can begin exploring more advanced strategies that may give your midlife metabolism an extra boost.

Intermittent Fasting

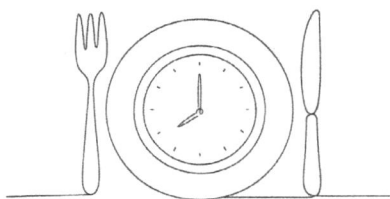

A Midlife Metabolism Reset

Many women are curious about intermittent fasting, and it's worth exploring. When done well, it can offer real benefits for midlife health. Research shows it may offer proven anti-aging benefits, from improving metabolic health and reducing inflammation to boosting insulin sensitivity and even supporting cellular repair through a process called autophagy. This approach can also be beneficial for maintaining a healthy weight, or even as a supportive weight-loss tool during menopause when metabolism often slows and hormonal shifts make balance more challenging.

Now, I know this might seem to contradict what I've said earlier about eating every 3 or 4 hours to support steady blood sugar and hormone health. But it's important to explore fasting, because many people are experiencing real benefits. The key is understanding *when* and *how* to use it, especially in midlife when our bodies are already under hormonal stress. It's not about deprivation. It's about giving your body strategic breaks and tuning in to what it really needs.

Fasting works by giving your digestion a rest. After about 12 to 16 hours of not eating, your body switches from burning stored glucose to burning fat for fuel, producing ketones. This gentle metabolic shift can improve focus, reduce cravings, support weight loss, and lower inflammation. It's like a reset button for your metabolism, especially helpful in midlife when insulin resistance becomes more common.

Fasting also activates autophagy, your body's natural house-cleaning system, which clears damaged cells and boosts repair. This can support gut health, improve energy, reduce bloating, and even sharpen your mind.

But, and this is important, if you're deep in the throes of menopause with fatigue, sleep issues, or extreme hormone fluctuations, fasting might actually add stress to your body. I know it did for me. At that time, I needed nourishment, consistency, and rest more than anything else. Only once I felt stronger did intermittent fasting become a supportive tool. Through trial and error, I discovered that the 16:8 rhythm works well for me, and it's a pattern I still follow today.

When it comes to fasting, there isn't a one-size-fits-all approach. Think of it like trying on different outfits until you find the one that feels right. Some women start gently with a 12:12 rhythm, where you fast for 12 hours (most of it while you sleep) and eat a healthy, balanced diet during the other twelve. Others extend that window into 14:10 or 16:8, choosing to eat within an 8 or 10-hour window that suits their lifestyle. A few experiments with the 5:2 approach, where you eat normally 5 days a week and keep calories lighter on 2 days. And then there are the more advanced styles, like alternate-day fasting or even occasional 24-hour fasts, though those can feel intense at midlife and need extra care. The point isn't to pick the "right" method, but to find what works with your body's rhythms, your energy, and your stage of life. What feels supportive and sustainable for you is always the best choice, rather than simply following what your girlfriend is doing.

If you're curious to try it, start gently. Begin with a 12-hour overnight fast and gradually extend by an hour each week. I recommend not going beyond 16 hours regularly. Why? Because after that point, fasting can become a stressor for your body, especially if your nervous system, hormones, or adrenals are already under pressure. Fasting too long can elevate cortisol, slow metabolism, disrupt sleep, and backfire by increasing cravings and fatigue later in the day. You want your body to feel safe, not starved. Instead, use fasting as a flexible tool. Start by trying it a few times a week rather than daily. Monitor your energy, sleep, and mood to see how your body responds.

When you do fast, make your eating window count. Focus on nutrient-dense meals with plenty of protein, fiber, and healthy fats. Personally, I find skipping breakfast and having a high-protein meal around eleven a.m. works best. But again, listen to your body. When I was navigating the rougher waters of menopause, fasting made things worse. Now that I'm through the other side, it's a helpful tool, but I still don't push beyond 16 hours. If I notice fatigue creeping in, I shift back to eating more regularly, which helps keep my energy stable. Fasting isn't a magic fix, but when timed right, it can be a powerful ally.

So, here's your new mantra: "Heal first. Fast later." Because when your blood sugar is steady, your hormones have a chance to recalibrate. This means your cravings should ease, and your body can release the weight it no longer needs to hold onto.

Quick tip:

Remember, this is about sustainably nourishing your body through this major life transition. Start small, maybe by upgrading your breakfast, and notice how you feel. Some women find they need more protein earlier in the day, others discover adding healthy fats to an afternoon snack stops that 5 p.m. eat-everything-in-sight frenzy.

Think of each meal as an opportunity to support your body, use your hand as a guide for portion size, and focus on protein, fiber, and healthy fats. You'll be laying a strong foundation for long-term health and vitality in no time. Whether you're vegetarian, paleo, gluten-free, or somewhere joyfully in between, these principles can be adapted to fit your life.

CHAPTER 11

Hydration to Thrive

"Water is life and clean water means health."

– AUDREY HEPBURN

Here's something that surprised me when I first hit my midlife wall: the decline of estrogen levels during perimenopause changes how our bodies manage water, making it easier to become depleted without even realizing it. Yep, just one more plot twist in the perimenopause journey!

This hormonal shift means our cells don't hold on to water as efficiently, making proper hydration essential, not just for energy and digestion, but for joint health, skin elasticity, mental clarity, and even hormone balance. But it's also so easy to overlook when you're busy, distracted, or juggling work, relationships, sleep struggles, and the general chaos of life. Reaching for a glass of water isn't always at the top of your mind. But trust me, this small habit can make a big difference.

I'll be honest: I thought I was doing all the right things. I was drinking smoothies, fresh juices, and (way too much) coffee. But I rarely drank just water unless I was working out or in the sauna. I avoided it during long client sessions and classes because, let's face it, who has time to sip water and for constant bathroom breaks when you're teaching back-to-back? Then came the brain fog, the crushing fatigue, and the hot flashes that felt like someone had turned on an internal heater. I was exhausted, and it wasn't just hormones. I was seriously dehydrated. Once I started tracking my intake, I realized I was barely drinking one liter a day. No wonder my energy was tanking!

Hydration quenches thirst. It also supports your brain, joints, digestion, and hormone transport. Since adult female bodies are made up of about 55% water, maintaining that balance becomes critical. Every cell in your body needs water to function properly, especially when hormones are shifting, temperature regulation is on high alert, and you're losing extra fluid through sweating.

Research shows that most midlife women should aim for 0.5 to 1 ounce of water per pound of body weight daily. So, if you weigh around 150 pounds, that amounts to about 2.2 to 4.4 liters per day, and even more if you're exercising, experiencing hot flashes, or living in a warm climate.

Fun fact: Each hot flash can cause you to lose up to 8 ounces of water!

Starting the day with warm water can be especially soothing. It's gentler on digestion than cold water, helps stimulate circulation, encourages healthy bowel movements, and helps calm the nervous system, which is often under extra strain in midlife. This simple ritual grounds you and sets a steady tone for the day ahead. Adding a pinch of Himalayan or sea salt or a squeeze of lemon can help with absorption and electrolyte balance. And if you're someone who forgets to drink, try habit-stacking, like sipping a glass of warm water while your coffee brews or keeping a water bottle in every room. Trust me, when you hydrate properly, everything improves energy, focus, skin, digestion, and even your cravings often settle down. Think of water as the simplest, most effective "supplement" you can give yourself during menopause.

Hydration Hack

Staying hydrated can feel like just another chore when your mind is already juggling hot flashes, work deadlines, and figuring out where you left your glasses. Here's the trick that made a difference for me: I gave up plastic bottles (more on that in a moment) and invested in three reliable 750ml stainless steel bottles. One stays in my car, one on my desk, and one at my Pilates studio. I fill them all each morning like my own little hydration squad. By the end of the day, if they're empty, I know I've done right by my body.

Plastics, Water Quality, and Hormones

Now, let's talk about plastics. Once I found out that cheap plastic bottles—yes, even the ones labeled "BPA-free"—mess with our already fragile hormonal balance, they were out. Many plastics release hormone-disrupting chemicals like BPS and BPF, especially when left in the sun or reused over time. And frankly, my hormones don't need any more drama. Stainless steel and glass bottles have become my go-to since then. Using them feels like a small daily act of self-respect.

And while we're at it, let's talk about the water going into those bottles. Drinking filtered water is essential. Tap water can carry a cocktail of chemicals, heavy metals, and residues, like chlorine, fluoride, and even traces of pharmaceutical drugs. When your hormones are already trying to find their new midlife groove, the last thing you need is extra toxins sneaking in with every sip.

Choosing filtered water is one of the simplest, most powerful ways you can reduce your body's toxic load. It also just tastes better, and we're far more likely to drink enough when it tastes clean and fresh.

One of my clients, Rebecca, a full-time high school teacher, was constantly battling headaches, migraines, and afternoon slumps. She admitted she avoided drinking water to reduce bathroom breaks between classes. She also drank coffee throughout her day to help with her afternoon fatigue. So, we came up with a hydration strategy that worked for her teaching blocks and included herbal teas and water-rich lunches. Within a couple of weeks, her headaches cut in half, there were hardly any more migraines, and she'd stopped hitting the 3 p.m. wall.

It's all about finding a rhythm that fits your life. Try starting your morning with a big glass of water before your coffee or tea (trust me; your body will thank you). I start the day with warm water and a pinch of Himalayan salt before detox tea. Keep your bottle nearby and sip steadily throughout the day. If plain water bores you, toss in some cucumber slices, lemon wedges, mint leaves, or a few berries to jazz it up. Herbal teas count, too, especially calming blends like chamomile or mint if stress is riding shotgun.

One of the simplest ways to check if you're staying well hydrated is to take a peek at your pee. Sounds basic, but your urine is a great hydration barometer. If it's clear or a pale straw color, you're likely drinking enough water. But if it's darker yellow, or worse—heading into orange territory—that's a clear sign your body's crying out for more fluids. Staying hydrated is important to help manage hot flashes, support digestion, prevent constipation, and keep your skin and joints supple. So, keep a bottle of water handy, and make sipping throughout the day a habit.

And don't forget the magic of electrolytes. As our hormones shift, so does our ability to retain key minerals like magnesium and potassium. Eating water-rich foods can help here, too. Cucumber, celery, watermelon, oranges, and strawberries are yummy hydration support.

What I've seen again and again is how hydration can subtly transform everything. Sleep improves, energy levels stabilize, hot flashes become less intense. Even cravings reduce. It's not a magic pill, but it comes close. And the best part? You just need a bottle or two and the willingness to check in with your body a bit more mindfully. Hydration is about showing up for yourself, one sip at a time.

Menopause and Alcohol

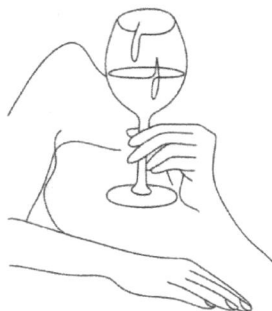

Let's talk about why that glass of wine might be doing more harm now. I get asked all the time (usually with a hopeful smirk), "Does my evening gin and tonic count as hydration?" Sadly, the answer is no. Alcohol dehydrates. It draws water out of your cells, puts pressure on your liver and kidneys, and leaves you feeling way worse. And during menopause, those effects can feel even more intense.

I used to enjoy a glass of full-bodied red wine, believing the antioxidants would boost my health and help me relax. But somewhere in my late forties, something changed. What once felt like a relaxing ritual started waking me up at two a.m., drenched in sweat with my heart racing. The next day, I'd wake up puffy, irritable, and sluggish. I blamed stress at first, until I realized my body simply couldn't handle alcohol anymore. Here's why: As estrogen declines, so does your body's ability to process alcohol. Estrogen helps regulate how the liver breaks down toxins, including alcohol. With less estrogen, the same drink hits harder and lingers longer. Add in a slower metabolism and shifts in body composition, and it's no wonder one glass now feels like three.

Alcohol also messes with your blood sugar, spikes cortisol, disrupts melatonin, and sends your circadian rhythm into chaos. That glass of wine might help you unwind in the moment, but hours later, it's often the reason you're staring at the ceiling, overheating, and feeling anxious in the dark.

Then there's the unnecessary calorie load. Empty, non-nutritive, and often underestimated. A large glass of wine can sneak in over 200 calories. Multiply that by a few glasses a week, and it adds up quickly, impacting everything from weight to mood to energy levels.

Now, this isn't about going teetotal, unless you want to. But it is about getting curious. If alcohol is leaving you feeling more drained than delighted, it might be time to reassess in an act of self-care. Many women I work with take a break, and the improvements often speak for themselves: better sleep, less bloating, clearer thinking, and more stable moods.

If you choose to drink, small shifts help. Choose clear spirits like gin or vodka with soda and citrus, instead of sugary mixers. Never drink on an empty stomach. Pair your drink with protein and healthy fats to help buffer blood sugar spikes. And yes, drink a full glass of water between alcoholic beverages. It's not glamorous but waking up clear-headed and fresh is worth it. Check in with your why. Are you drinking for joy, or has it become a coping tool? Is it a habit or a conscious choice? Could you decompress with something else, like a walk, bath, or laugh with a friend?

Menopause is a chance to rewrite old rules. Your "fussy" body is just telling you what it needs and what it no longer tolerates. You're still fun and fabulous. And let's be real, these days, the alcohol-free options are just as chic and way more energizing. A fancy glass of sparkling water with lime or a delicious alcohol-free spirit can also feel indulgent, without regret, hangover, or night sweats.

Caffeine

While we're on the subject of drinks, we can't skip coffee. Yes, I love it, too. But if you're experiencing hot flashes, anxiety, heart palpitations, insomnia, or that wired-but-exhausted feeling, caffeine could make it worse. It stimulates your adrenals, which are already taxed by midlife stress, and can push your nervous system further into overdrive. No need to go cold turkey (don't panic), but cutting back or switching to decaf can make a noticeable difference. If you choose decaf, pick a water-processed one. It's free of the harsh chemicals used in conventional decaffeination. That way, you still get the taste, without adding more stress to your system.

Make sure you never drink coffee on an empty stomach. Have it after breakfast, not first thing. Even swapping one cup for a calming herbal tea or matcha can help keep your energy levels stable throughout the day. That is, after all, what this is all about: slowly and gently shifting into a more stable approach to nourishing. It'll take time, but every little step and sustained habit change counts. Pat yourself on the back. You've come pretty far already.

Essential Supplements for Midlife Wellness

Midlife is a time of incredible hormonal, physical, and emotional change, and your nutrient needs shift right along with it. Of course, nourishing food should always be your first go-to. But absorbing nutrients from food gets trickier as we age. Stress depletes key micronutrients, like vitamins and minerals faster than we realize. Medications, digestive changes, and even chronic low-level inflammation can interfere with absorption.

That's where smart, targeted supplementation can help. I've found that the right vitamins complement my nourishing diet. They give me extra energy, help me stay clear-headed, and support my hormones so I feel more resilient. You can also ask your doctor for blood tests to see where you might be deficient, especially in micronutrients like the B vitamins that are so important for energy. Vitamin D is another one to check, as it's often low in midlife women and is critical for bone strength, mood, and immune health.

To make it easy, I put my vitamins together with my hormones each Sunday in a seven-day, day-and-night pill container. I keep it in the drawer beside my bed, which makes it simple to stay consistent. It's also a lifesaver on those brain fog days when I'm most likely to forget.

So, while we aim to eat well, I see supplements as a safety net. They act as a steady backup that helps fill in the gaps and give my body a little extra love where it needs it most.

Targeted Nutrient Support

Multivitamins

If you're someone who only wants to take one pill a day, a good-quality multivitamin can be a simple, effective way to cover your nutritional bases. It should include bioavailable forms of key nutrients your body can readily absorb and use. Look for one that contains methylated B vitamins (like B12 and folate), vitamin D3, magnesium (in gentle forms like citrate or glycinate), zinc, selenium, and vitamin K2 for bone and hormone support.

If you're dealing with fatigue, sleeping problems, sore muscles, body aches, poor recovery, low mood, or brain fog, these nutrients could be part of the missing puzzle piece. But, while a well-rounded multivitamin isn't a magic bullet, it's a simple way to give your midlife body the extra support it may be craving. Think of it as a daily reset button for your system.

Magnesium

Magnesium is one of the most common deficiencies in midlife. It's also one of the most important ones to correct. As we age, stress, poor sleep, and hormone shifts can deplete our stores, leading to muscle tension, anxiety, headaches, restless legs, or disrupted sleep. This calming mineral supports your nervous system, helps balance hormones, aids digestion, and even improves bone density.

I often recommend magnesium glycinate for deep relaxation and better sleep, and magnesium citrate for gentle digestive support. Many of my clients notice a real difference within just a few days, from fewer muscle cramps and faster recovery to better sleep and a greater sense of calm.

Ashwagandha

This adaptogen is traditionally used in Ayurvedic medicine for menopause symptoms. It may help your body respond to stress better, regulate cortisol, lower anxiety, brain fog and hot flashes, improve mood, and support thyroid and sleep. Many women say they feel more emotionally stable and grounded after adding it to their diet. While researchers are still investigating how ashwagandha interacts with your body, there are some studies showing it may have an impact on levels of reproductive hormones, including estrogen and FSH. Changes in these can be at the core of symptoms during perimenopause and menopause.

Melatonin

Your "sleep hormone" also has powerful antioxidants and anti-inflammatory benefits. Melatonin levels naturally decline with age, and the drop often accelerates during perimenopause and menopause. This is partly due to changes in the brain's pineal gland (where melatonin is produced), along with hormonal shifts like declining estrogen and progesterone that disrupt its natural rhythm. If you're struggling to fall asleep, waking in the early hours, or feeling out of sync, melatonin can help reset your internal clock. It's gentle but effective and worth discussing with your health care provider if sleep becomes elusive.

Vitamin D3

You may know vitamin D3 as the "sun vitamin," as levels in the body can be linked to sun exposure. It's essential for bone strength, immune function, hormone balance, and mood. Vitamin D3 levels often drop with age, especially if you're not getting enough regular sun exposure or if your body's ability to absorb vitamin D has declined. If you're feeling achy, flat, and/or are getting sick more often, it might be time to have your levels checked. I get a doctor-prescribed D3 dose once a month. It's super easy and makes a difference.

Calcium

You may not have thought about your calcium intake much until now, but it becomes important after menopause. Lower estrogen levels increase your risk of bone loss. Food, weight-bearing exercise, and supplementation are your go-to. If you take supplements, make sure they are spread out, as the body can only absorb so much in one go. Aim for whole food sources like sardines (with the bones), tahini, sesame seeds, almonds, or leafy greens. For best absorption, pair calcium with magnesium and vitamin D, as they work together to support bone strength and prevent brittle bones down the track.

Zinc

This essential mineral helps hormone regulation, immune function, skin repair, and healing. Plus, it supports healthy hair and strong nails (which many of us notice thinning during menopause). I take a prescription 50 mg zinc sulfate capsules every night before bed, and I keep an eye on my levels with regular blood tests. Zinc can be easily depleted by stress, illness, or certain medications, so it's worth checking if you're feeling rundown or your skin and nails need extra support.

Selenium

A powerful antioxidant that's essential in midlife, as it supports thyroid health, immune defense, and hormone balance. Eggs, meat, grains, and cereals contain selenium, although selenium levels depend on the animal's or plant's intake from soil. These can be quite low in countries such as New Zealand, Australia, and parts of Europe. Shellfish, sardines, or tuna can cover your daily selenium needs. If you're vegetarian or having a plant-based day, supplements or one to two Brazil nuts offer a simple solution.

B Vitamins

A combination of B6, B12, and folate (also called B9) is essential for your body. The trio supports energy production, metabolism, mental clarity, mood, nervous system health, and even hair health. B12 boosts energy, focus, mood, and nerve health. If your diet is mostly plant-based, you might need more of it since it's mainly found in animal products. As we age, we also absorb less of it, especially if stomach acid levels decrease or digestion becomes impaired. Personally, I take a regular high-dose vitamin B12, and I've found it really helps to support my energy.

Vitamin B6 can help regulate mood, improve sleep quality, and potentially lessen the severity of hot flashes. It plays a crucial role in producing neurotransmitters like serotonin, which can help with mood swings and depression, and melatonin, connecting it to sleep regulation. Folate may help reduce hot flashes, support cognitive function, and promote bone health. A vitamin B-complex may be beneficial if you're experiencing a variety of symptoms, especially fatigue and low mood.

Iron

Iron plays a vital role in oxygen transport, influencing brain function and physical stamina. Low iron levels can cause tiredness, brain fog, breathlessness, dizziness, fainting, and a general feeling of exhaustion. Even if your periods have become lighter or stopped, your iron stores, both short-term and long-term, may still be low, especially if you have a history of heavy bleeding, digestive issues, or low intake (such as from a plant-based diet).

If fatigue persists, despite rest and proper nutrition, it's important to have your iron levels checked. Supplementing with a highly bioavailable iron supplement, preferably with vitamin C, to enhance absorption, and avoiding coffee can help replenish your short-term stores. Additionally, making a sustained effort to improve absorption or take supplements will help rebuild long-term stores, which can take months. Don't delay seeking medical advice.

Vitamin C

Known for its immune-boosting properties, vitamin C is also a potent antioxidant. It helps shield the body's cells from free radical damage, which can slow aging and prevent chronic diseases. It also plays a crucial role in adrenal health and collagen production. This is especially important during menopause when stress can hit harder, and skin naturally loses elasticity. While many fruits are rich in vitamin C, you might not realize that it's also found in red and green peppers, broccoli, Brussels sprouts, cabbage, cauliflower, potatoes (especially baked ones), tomatoes, kale, spinach, and chili peppers. Vitamin C further enhances iron absorption and can help increase energy levels. I love taking it in powdered form with water first thing in the morning; it feels like a refreshing and nourishing way to start my day.

Amino Acids

Amino acids are the building blocks of protein, which means they support your muscles, brain chemicals, and hormones, all of which need extra care during midlife. As estrogen declines, we naturally lose muscle mass more easily and may notice slower recovery, low mood, or brain fog. If you get enough from complete animal sources such as meat, poultry, fish, eggs, dairy, soy products (like tofu and tempeh), quinoa, and buckwheat, or from incomplete plant sources, such as nuts, you won't need to worry. But if your protein intake isn't steady or your digestion isn't optimal, a supplement of essential amino acids can help fill the gap. They support muscle maintenance, tissue repair, and even neurotransmitter production, which is vital for mood, motivation, and memory.

Prebiotics

If you're not getting enough fiber-rich foods daily (hello, busy life), a prebiotic supplement can help nourish your gut bacteria. These usually contain fibers like inulin, FOS (fructooligosaccharides), or partially hydrolyzed guar gum, which feed your good microbes. Just start slow, because too much too soon can cause bloating. I often recommend introducing prebiotics gradually alongside a quality probiotic to support gut balance, digestion, and even hormone detox pathways. But chances are you're eating prebiotics without realizing it, as they are found in many foods such as bananas, apples, berries, asparagus, onions, garlic, Jerusalem artichokes, dandelion greens, leeks, beans, oats, barley, wheat bran, and whole grain products.

Probiotics

A good probiotic can strengthen your gut microbiome, support hormone clearance, improve digestion, and boost mood and immunity. Look for strains like Lactobacillus and Bifidobacterium with at least several billion CFUs. If you're new to probiotics, start slowly and observe how your digestion and energy levels respond. For even better results, pair them with prebiotic-rich foods, such as yogurt, sauerkraut, kombucha, kimchi, kefir, or pickles, or use a gentle prebiotic supplement to help those good bugs thrive.

I've even had my microbiome tested. Interestingly, the probiotic I was taking wasn't the missing link after all. Now I focus on variety, choosing different strains and mixing up the probiotics I buy to give my gut the widest support possible.

Vitamin E

This powerful antioxidant helps reduce oxidative stress and supports hormone balance, skin health, and immune function. It's also being researched for assisting with hot flashes, sleep quality, mood stability, and potentially bone health, making it invaluable during midlife when your body needs extra support.

Maca Root

Also known as Peruvian ginseng, this potent root helps your body balance its hormones. Traditionally used to boost energy, stamina, and mood, many women in midlife also notice an increase in libido and overall vitality. It's beneficial during hormonal shifts, providing gentle support without disrupting your body's natural rhythms. When I was experiencing severe menopausal symptoms, I found that taking maca daily, either as a teaspoon of powder blended into my smoothies or as a capsule, helped ease my fatigue.

Omega-3 Fatty Acids

Found in fatty fish, flaxseed, and supplements, omega-3s reduce inflammation, support heart health, boost mood, and aid joint and brain function. Since all of these are key processes for you in midlife and for your long-term health, it's one of the most important supplements to take. If you're not eating oily fish often, a high-quality supplement should be on your list of nutrition options.

Methylated Folate (not folic acid)

Studies suggest that methylated folate can help relieve some menopause symptoms by easing hot flashes, reducing the risk of osteoporosis, and protecting against age-related cognitive decline. Many standard multivitamins still contain folic acid (the synthetic version), which doesn't work well for everyone, especially if you have a common MTHFR gene variant. The activated, bioavailable form that your body can use is called methylated folate.

Liver Detox Complex

By the time we hit midlife, our livers have been working hard behind the scenes for decades, processing everything from hormonal shifts, alcohol, medications, and environmental toxins to stress and processed foods. Now, with fluctuating estrogen levels and a body that's not as forgiving as it once was, your liver needs some extra support.

Your liver plays an essential role in breaking down hormones, especially estrogen. When it's sluggish or overworked, excess hormones can accumulate and cause symptoms like bloating, irritability, heavy periods, fatigue, and weight gain around the middle. A supported liver can help clear this hormonal "clutter," leaving you feeling lighter, clearer, and more balanced.

That's why I believe in daily, gentle liver support and consistent care to help this organ do its job. I like to take a liver detox formula that combines powerful herbs and nutrients to support hormone metabolism and everyday detoxification.

Some of the best ingredients to look for are:

- Milk Thistle Extract is known for supporting liver cell regeneration and detox capacity.

- Dandelion Root promotes bile flow to help your body eliminate waste more efficiently.

- Artichoke Extract assists with fat metabolism and digestion, especially helpful if your gallbladder is sluggish.

- Curcumin C3 Complex is a concentrated form of turmeric with anti-inflammatory benefits.

- Ginger and Biopterin (black pepper extract) enhances nutrient absorption and soothes digestion.

If I've had a glass of wine, rich food, or a long, stressful day, I'll take an extra capsule before bed to help my liver process the additional load.

Gentle Daily Detox Habits

You don't need to overhaul your life to show your liver some love. These simple daily rituals can make a huge difference:

- Start the day with warm lemon water or apple cider vinegar in water to stimulate digestion.

- Take a moment to check in on your stress levels and remember to breathe. Deep, conscious breathing can be one of your body's most powerful natural detoxifiers.

- Add cruciferous vegetables like broccoli, cauliflower, and kale to your meals. They're fantastic for estrogen clearance.

- Drink plenty of filtered water to flush out toxins.

- Eat fiber-rich foods like chia seeds, flaxseeds, leafy greens, and berries to support elimination.

- Move your body. Even gentle movement helps detoxification via the lymphatic system.

- Cut back on alcohol, processed foods, and excess sugar. They all place strain on your liver.

Supportive Herbal Teas

Sometimes the simplest rituals bring the most potent results. A warm cup of herbal tea can be more than just hydration; it can soothe stress, support digestion, calm your nervous system, and gently help your body balance hormones. Here are some of my midlife favorites, grouped by their benefits:

Licorice Root

Naturally sweet and adaptogenic, licorice supports adrenal health and gives a gentle lift without caffeine. Helpful for afternoon fatigue and staying focused without feeling wired.

Ashwagandha (as tea or tincture)

An adaptogen that supports your stress response while gently boosting resilience. Great paired with cinnamon or cardamom for a warming twist.

Dandelion Root or Leaf

A natural liver tonic that supports gentle detox and estrogen clearance. Helps relieve bloating and sluggish digestion. Best enjoyed after meals. My personal favorite is a detox tea made from dandelion and milk thistle with a squeeze of lemon, a simple blend that offers gentle, natural cleansing support.

Peppermint

Calms the digestive tract and reduces bloating or gas. Refreshing and slightly cooling, perfect after meals or when hot flashes hit.

Chamomile

Soothes the nervous system and supports restful sleep. Perfect for winding down in the evening, especially if anxiety or overthinking creeps in.

Lemon Balm

A calming herb that supports mood, stress relief, and emotional balance. A favorite for the early evening or when your mind needs a gentle reset.

Red Clover

Rich in natural phytoestrogens, red clover is known to support hormonal equilibrium and ease hot flashes or night sweats during perimenopause and menopause.

Quick Tip:

I keep a little "tea drawer" stocked with a few favorites. In the afternoon, instead of automatically reaching for a snack or another coffee, I pause and ask, "What do I need right now?" Sometimes, it's dandelion for my belly. Sometimes, licorice for energy. Sometimes, chamomile so I can breathe and settle. In my book, tea isn't just tea; it's presence, practice, and powerful self-care in a cup.

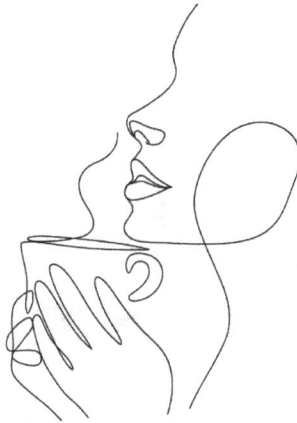

Test, Track, and Trust

Not every supplement will work for every woman. Some of us tolerate dairy; some of us don't. Some women need extra iron; others don't. The key is to test, track, and trust yourself. Keep a symptom journal, get blood tests done regularly, and work with a health care professional who listens.

I've personally tried many of these over the years. Some helped a little. Others were life changing. What matters is tuning in and staying curious. Midlife can be a beautiful, powerful turning point for you. And with the right nutritional support, you can feel clear, strong, and vibrant again.

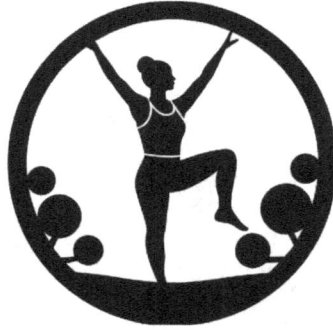

Pillar Three – Move For Life

"I do as I feel, and I like to stay active and be around people. I still want to keep moving. If I sat down, I think I'd just give up."

– TONI STAHL, WHO WORKS OUT REGULARLY AT AGE 100!

Toni's words remind us that movement is less about age or ability and more about intention and attitude.

Your mindset matters when it comes to all five pillars of the Vitality Blueprint, and this applies to movement, as well. When we're in survival mode, many of us stick to what we know has worked before. Often, that is workouts that leave us drenched in sweat and riding an endorphin high. I also used to believe the harder I pushed, the better I'd feel. Intense exercise was my go-to stress relief and letting go of that approach felt like losing a part of myself. But as our bodies change, we need to adapt. Now, I find lifting something heavy utterly satisfying, both in everyday life and during workouts. It makes me feel strong and capable. Feeling confident in my body is empowering in a whole new way.

CHAPTER 12

Movement with Intention

"The body will become better at whatever you do, or don't do. If you don't move, your body will make you better at not moving."

BEN MEDDER

It's a gentle reminder that our bodies adapt to what we ask of them. Even the smallest, lightest movements send a signal that we want to stay flexible, strong, and alive in our skin. Regular movement supports recovery and keeps the whole system humming.

I learned about movement at an early age, growing up on a wild family farm with five siblings. So, movement has always been an integral part of my life. It used to be how I boosted my energy and felt like myself. But over the years, I've learned that different seasons call for different approaches to movement. Shaped by my upbringing and healing life experiences, I also believe strength goes beyond the physical.

In my thirties, after a traumatic ectopic pregnancy that left me weak and frail, I rebuilt my strength with the help of a personal trainer. This new gym-based approach to movement left me not only stronger but also calmer and more confident. The results I experienced were so inspiring they sparked a new path for me, ultimately leading me to train as a personal trainer and Pilates instructor. I wanted to help others experience that same transformation through greater presence.

I firmly believe that strength is about showing up and listening deeply, even when your body's messages and signals feel uncomfortable. It's about resilience. Sometimes, just showing up is enough.

This chapter will help you find a new connection and approach to movement. This stage of life is about smart and aligned workout choices. Movement that empowers you as part of your daily life. Exercise bursts that boost your energy. Making mindful choices to align your posture and cultivate both inner and outer strength. The key is tuning in and responding with care and consideration (your days of gung-ho powering through are done).

As your hormone levels decline, your joints may feel stiffer, your body might ache, and sleep can become more fragile, leaving you tired and with less mental bandwidth. Additionally, your stress tolerance drops, and your body responds differently to input, even if it's movement. It becomes more challenging to build muscles and strength. Your body now needs a supportive, mindful approach to exercise that incorporates rhythm. Most importantly, it needs you to choose movement that energizes rather than depletes.

Supporting Factors

Working out what works when and adapting to your body's changing needs, also means harnessing anything that can support you. These factors will help maximize what you get out of your exercise and keep you going, even on days you may not feel like it. Too often we think of exercise as something we "have to do," whether it's to fit into clothes, reach a certain dress size, burn off a hamburger and fries, or tick a box on someone else's idea of what's "good for us." But having that mindset pulls us away from the joy of moving.

While those reasons may feel motivating in the moment, the truth is they're rooted in what we think we *should* do rather than what we truly want. The real shift happens when you focus on enjoyment and positive reinforcement. This helps you not only enjoy your workout but also feel the benefits in your day-to-day life, guiding you back to listening to your body and your own inner wisdom.

Choosing what works for you now includes listening, learning what works for you, and a promise to yourself that you are doing it for all the right reasons: claiming back agency, vitality, and confidence. A good starting point can be to sit with yourself for a moment and think about positive experiences you have had with exercise in the past. Oftentimes, we can reframe the setting or conditions enough to still reap the benefits and have a great time while doing it.

As an example, some exercises can be reframed as stepping stones to reach the parts you enjoy. Diana discovered reformer Pilates after a back injury left her unable to do her favorite long-distance runs in her twenties. She'd previously tried mat Pilates at a gym and gotten bored within five minutes of lying on her mat and activating muscles. But when a dancer friend recommended she try a reformer Pilates class, that first class had her hooked. She soon returned to running but kept a lifelong habit of reformer Pilates to support her through injuries, pregnancies, and shifting needs. While you don't have to become an instructor to enjoy it, *watch out!* it may just hook you, too.

Movement Motivators

Figuring out what works for you and what you will stick with comes down to what motivates you. Motivational factors can be defined as intrinsic (internal) and extrinsic (external). Intrinsic motivators feel good from the inside out. You feel it in the lift of your mood and the calm that follows movement. You notice it as you master new skills and grow stronger. There's that extra spark of vitality, the quiet pride of showing up for yourself, and the deep, easy sleep that follows.

Extrinsic motivators come from the world around you. They include managing your weight, improving health markers, and feeling more confident in your appearance. They might come from social support, a workout buddy, or a class community. Sometimes, it's the simple encouragement or recognition that keeps you showing up. Take a seat and think. What exercise have you enjoyed in the past and why? Perhaps those HIIT sessions were your jam because they release a ton of endorphins, lowering your stress and anxiety levels? Maybe you enjoy recharging by yourself and hiking in nature? Understanding what keeps you coming back will go a long way toward making exercise feel less like a chore and more like a pleasurable experience.

Most of us are motivated by multiple factors. For example, scheduling a workout with a friend may tick several extrinsic factors, as you may enjoy the social connection, feel compelled not to miss a session, boost your body image and long-term health, while also feeling more energetic and in a good mood. If you are more introverted or like to recharge by being by yourself, a walk-run in nature may tick better boxes for you, as it will probably hit most of the intrinsic factors.

For your new movement habits to stick, it's a good idea to try a range of different exercise activities over several weeks and see what leaves you feeling best. On some days, a lap around your local park after breakfast might feel perfect. On others, when even leaving the house feels like a chore, a few stretches or a gentle Pilates session at home could be just what you need.

Let's have a look at the different types of exercise you should start incorporating for maximum long-term vitality.

Benefits of Outdoor Exercise

The most nourishing ways to move in midlife are those that support your nervous system: barefoot beach walks to clear your mind, kayaking on a lake before the busy day, cycling leisurely along the foreshore or through the countryside, and quiet strolls through green spaces that feel like a deep exhale. When you move your body outdoors, especially in the morning light, you're sending positive signals to your brain while getting your steps in at the same time.

The first step in supporting your nervous system during exercise is exposure to sunlight, which helps regulate your circadian rhythm. Spending ten to twenty minutes in natural morning light can help reset your circadian rhythm and improve your sleep, energy, and hormone production. Morning light also stimulates cortisol appropriately (giving you that energy boost) while helping to kick-start melatonin production in the evening, leading to better sleep. It's one of the simplest, most underrated wellness tools we have, and it's free.

Try scheduling your exercise outside whenever possible or simply go for a slow walk for a winning combination. Moving your body outdoors helps regulate your nervous system, balancing your fight-or-flight response with the rest-and-digest response. When your nervous system often feels stuck in "on" mode during midlife, this kind of regulation is essential.

Healing Movement

Moving your body in green spaces does more than boost fitness. It lowers blood pressure, calms cortisol levels, eases anxiety, and even strengthens your immune function. The Japanese call this healing practice "forest bathing" or *shinrin-yoku*. It's simply walking in the forest and letting nature do its quiet magic. You can find your own version anywhere. A neighborhood path, a local park, or even your garden can become a healing space.

Let yourself slow down. Unplug from the constant ping of messages and text reminders. Leave the headphones at home. Let your senses wake up. Listen to the crunch of gravel under your shoes. The smell of eucalyptus or fresh grass. Feel the warmth of sunlight on your cheeks, the gentle rustle of wind in the trees, or the birdsong overhead. These are nature's reminders that your body is safe and grounded.

In midlife, life often feels demanding, yet your body is asking for calm. Stillness. Simplicity. This is where real healing begins.

Just remember to take it one session at a time. Try keeping track of your sessions and celebrate your progress along the way. Maybe treat yourself to a new pair of leggings or a yoga mat after twenty walks. Small rewards keep motivation high and help movement feel joyful, not forced.

Research also shows that one of the best ways to build cardiovascular health is by breaking movement into smaller bursts throughout the day. A gentle walk to and from work. Take the stairs instead of taking the elevator. A quick lap around the block all count. These short, regular bouts of activity are more realistic and more effective than forcing yourself through an exhausting one-hour workout when you're already tired.

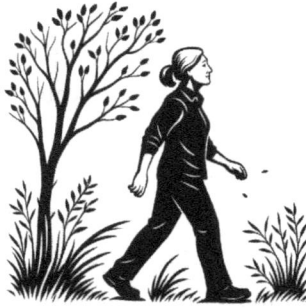

What matters most is that you keep moving, gently and consistently, in ways that make you feel alive.

Finding Your Sweet Spot

If you're wondering how to know whether you're moving "enough," there's a simple way to find out. It's all about balance. Moving with purpose but not pushing your body into stress.

In fitness terms, this balance relates to something called VO_2 max. It sounds complicated, but it just means how well your heart, lungs, and muscles work together when you exercise. Think of it as your body's engine power. For most midlife women, the sweet spot is cruising at about 60 to 70% of VO_2 max. At this pace, you build strength and stamina, improving metabolism, and tap into fat-burning without tipping your body into stress mode.

You don't need lab equipment to figure this out. Just use the "talk test." If your breathing is heavier but you can still hold a conversation, with a few pauses for air, you're right where you need to be. If you're gasping and can't speak, slow down a little.

For those of you who enjoy nerding out over numbers, most fitness watches estimate VO_2 max and give you heart rate zones. A simple way to check is by using your maximum heart rate, which is roughly 220 minus your age. From there, aim for about 60 to 70% of that number. For example, if you're 50, your maximum heart rate is around 170, so your target range is about 102 to 119 beats per minute.

Listen to Your Body

Whether you go by feel or by figures, the goal is the same: Pay attention to how you feel afterward. Energized? Slightly more mobile? More grounded in your body? That's progress. If you push too hard, you may end up crashing later in the day and undo your good work. Aim to finish your workout feeling refreshed, not wrung out. That's how you build consistency and keep movement joyful.

Some days, you'll feel strong and ready to move. Other days, not so much. Midlife is the time to tune into your body, pushing when energy is high. Rest when your body asks for it. This intuitive approach helps prevent burnout, supports hormonal balance, and keeps you coming back.

To build consistency, if you're new to exercising, start small. Two to three short sessions a week are enough to get started. Even ten to fifteen minutes count. That might mean one simple strength-based bodyweight session, one walk outdoors, and one dedicated day for stretching or mobility. You're laying the foundation and keeping things light and energizing.

Maximizing a focus on low-impact and high-benefit exercise keeps your routine sustainable and energizing. Walking, swimming, cycling, and rebounding are all gentle on your joints while still delivering cardiovascular, lymphatic, and mental health benefits. They help you stay active without adding physical stress.

Starting from Zero

If you're starting from scratch, don't despair. Take a deep breath and drop the pressure. You're not behind, even if your health has taken a backseat, and you haven't exercised in a while. You're exactly where you need to be, and starting now is brave. This is about rebuilding trust in your body first. You'll focus on creating strength and stability. Over time, you'll rebuild your energy from the ground up.

You can begin right where you are, in your own home and backyard. No frills. No fancy gear needed. Begin with gentle movements that feel safe and doable. This could be a ten-minute walk around the block, following a breath-led Pilates video on your living room floor, or quiet stretching before bed. The key is consistency. Small, repeatable actions make the biggest difference. Find what motivates you and make it easy to keep going.

Gearing Up

You don't need a gym membership or fancy equipment to get started, really. But investing in a few key pieces makes it easier to move. A good pair of supportive walking shoes that feel comfortable the moment you slip them on will help you prevent unnecessary soreness and injuries (more important now; trust me!). Running shoes can double up as walking and exercising shoes initially, especially with a bit of tread on the bottom to prevent slipping on wet days or unstable terrain.

A simple yoga mat can be used for functional exercise, Pilates, stretching, yoga, and even meditation. Keep it somewhere visible as a cue to move. Place your mat or shoes where they'll remind you to use them, like next to the bed in the morning, by the door, or perhaps place the mat on the kitchen table to remember that yesterday's you thought exercising would be a good idea today.

It helps to treat your movement like something worth preparing for. A high-quality water bottle can make hydration easy and intentional. Comfortable workout clothes that don't rub or restrict your movement makes a world of difference. Choose fabric that breathes, stretches, and moves with you so nothing gets in the way of how good it feels to move your body. These small investments become daily reminders that you matter, and your wellbeing is worth prioritizing.

How to Choose

Choosing the right exercise can feel confusing, especially when you're unlearning old habits. Many of us grew up believing that harder is better, that long cardio burns more fat, or that weights make you bulky. In midlife, those beliefs often backfire. You end up feeling tired, sore, or gaining weight despite all the effort.

This next stage is about working smarter. Swap long, hard cardio sessions with shorter, more balanced activities, like walking, Pilates, strength training, or low-impact intervals. This can transform how you feel, look, and recover.

The bottom line is that, in midlife, movement should make you feel stronger and more stable, never exhausted or burned out. Choose activities that build you up, not wear you down. This is your training for strength, clarity, energy, and mobility. Not just for now, but for decades to come.

With the right approach, you're doing much more than building muscle. You're regulating blood sugar, balancing hormones, supporting cognitive function, and boosting your metabolism. You're helping your body sleep more deeply, stabilize your mood, and manage stress more effectively. You're protecting your bone density and joint health. You're also preserving your strength and mobility that allow you to stay independent, active, and confident through every season of life.

Your Pick-and-Choose Movement Mix

- Short Bursts of Movement. Weave short bursts of movement throughout your day whenever you can. Take the stairs instead of the elevator, doing some push-ups against your kitchen counter while waiting for the kettle to boil, or balancing on one leg while brushing your teeth. These quick activities help build strength, improve mood, and energize you without causing cortisol spikes or draining your energy. If you enjoy them, extend to 15 to 30 minutes of mixed functional exercises. Consistent little bursts add up and keep your body happy without overdoing it.

- Functional Movements, Core, and Range of Motion. Years of sitting and daily habits can lead to stiffness and limited range of motion. Functional training uses everyday patterns, like squats or hinges, the movements that help you lift, reach, and twist, to help you move with ease and confidence. Yoga and Pilates both support this, but Pilates is specifically designed for core strength and functional alignment. Power yoga and reformer Pilates can also surprise you with their strength benefits.

- Strength Training. Building and maintaining muscle is vital at midlife. Resistance training with bands, lifting weights, or bodyweight exercises all work to protect bone health, boost metabolism, and prevent muscle loss. Two to three weight-bearing workouts each week can have a big impact, but even just one consistent workout helps. Just remember to listen to your body and take it easy when needed. Progress happens with patience.

- Moderate-Intensity Cardio. Choose movement that keeps your heart rate steady and manageable. Think brisk walking, relaxed cycling, kayaking, or swimming. Aim for about 150 minutes (which is only 30 minutes five days of the week) to maintain a healthy heart and regulate cortisol. This allows you to stay active without increasing stress hormones or losing muscle. Try weaving activities into your day. Keeping a jump rope nearby or your sneakers by the door makes it easy. Even a quick walk around the block can help build your fitness.

- High-Intensity Interval Training (HIIT). Short, well-timed bursts of effort followed by rest can help burn fat, preserve muscle, and support metabolism. If you're new to HIIT, keep sessions to around 20 minutes. If you're more experienced, limit the main workout to no more than 30 minutes, always allowing time for a proper warm-up and cool-down. These quick bursts of effort followed by rest can help you burn fat, preserve muscle, and keep cortisol levels under control. Start simply by adding intervals to your walks, like choosing a hilly trail or a staircase to naturally raise the intensity.

- Stretching and Mobility. Gentle mobility work keeps you flexible and pain-free. As your body begins to feel stiffer and postural habits become more ingrained, activities like stretching and mobility work, such as foam rolling, held stretches, or flowing yoga sessions, can help you regain better ranges of motion and experience less soreness. These practices also boost circulation, reduce stiffness, and support pelvic health, posture, and balance. Gentle Pilates or yoga sessions calm the nervous system and help shift your body out of "fight or flight" mode and into a state of calm and connection.

Quick Fix: Short Bursts of Movement

If you're new to exercise or have a busy life, fitting in more than a few minutes a day might seem ambitious, but don't lose hope. Short, intense training (SIT) of just two to three minutes several times a day can work wonders. It's similar to adding protein throughout your meals to stay fueled, instead of eating it all at once.

It may initially require you to think outside the box (and yes, wearing comfortable pants and tops help), but once you start, the benefits and positive effects will motivate you to keep going. Your energy, focus, and mood will improve, and you may even progress to longer sessions. Best of all, SIT lowers your risk of long-term diseases and effectively age-proofs your body through exercise snacking. It's also easier to stay consistent and avoid overdoing it. You'll finish energized, not exhausted. Sounds doable?

Here's how you do SIT:

- A minimum commitment to gain benefits might be just 3 one-minute exercise sessions a day.

- An intermediate commitment looks like 4 sessions of two minutes of SIT. Keep it up, and you'll soon want to extend.

- Maximum commitment is about 5 sessions of three minutes of SIT. At this point, you may like to add in a single ten-minute workout instead, whenever it suits you.

Exercise Examples

It's important to choose the activities you're most likely to stick with, while mixing things up and trying a few challenging exercises, as well. So, make sure you don't get stuck in a squat-only rut once you've built some momentum.

- Functional exercises. Stairs, squats, lunges (if your knees are okay), burpees, crab walk, side-to-side step.

- Cardio exercises. Jumping jacks, shadow boxing, mountain climbers, jump squats, high knees, fast feet, stair walks or runs, plank jacks.

- Core exercises. Mountain climbers, superman, kneeling side plank, plank hold with alternating hand lift, bicycle crunches, sit-ups, 100s, pointer dog, high plank hold.

- Upper body strength. Push-ups (knees or wall), triceps dips (chair or desk), resistance band biceps curls standing, high to low plank, shoulder circles, chopping wood.

- Lower body strength. Wall sits, lunge pulses, glute bridges, single-leg deadlifts, single-leg stands, held lunges.

If you're new to training or working out in the office, start with modified versions at a low intensity. Focusing on functional patterns like squats, lunges, hinges, twists, pushes, pulls, and core movements. These compound exercises engage multiple muscle groups, giving you the best return on your time. Ideally, do 2 to 3 exercises during each SIT session and work just hard enough to feel a little energized but not overly puffed. You'll soon want to do more!

The best part is, you can do this every day and incorporate it into your existing routine. Think squats while brushing your teeth, benchtop push-ups while waiting for the kettle to boil, cycling between reading a work document to stay focused and alert.

Bonus Tip:

Add one stretching or breathwork snacks-ercize before bed. It'll help you signal to your nervous system to wind down. You'll sleep more deeply and wake up ready to move again.

CHAPTER 13

Building Strength and Resilience

"Feeling strong gives me the freedom to live life boldly.
Strength training isn't about perfection; it's about creating
a life without physical or mental limits."

– LUCI HARRISON, MIDLIFE COACH AND AUTHOR

Think of your body like a well-loved car: It needs regular maintenance, an oil change, and everything working together to perform at its best. During menopause, your "maintenance plan" for exercise becomes a balanced mix of strength training, mobility work, and daily movement. These are your tune-ups. They keep your engine (aka metabolism) running smoothly, your joints moving freely, your mind sharp, and your energy steady. Neglect the muscles, and much like skipping car services, things start to break down. You feel flatter, stiffer, and more tired, simply because your body is missing the proper support it now needs.

If you're still unsure about when to do what, here's a more detailed explanation of how to build each type of movement into your week. Exercise can be divided into categories.

Those that build strength.

Those that improve cardiovascular health.

And those that enhance function and posture.

Below, you'll find each exercise type listed with its most common forms, benefits, and ideal times to do them.

Why You Need to Build Strength

Muscle loss already starts sneaking in during our mid-thirties, long before most of us think about menopause. Without regular strength training, women can lose 3 to 8% of muscle mass each decade. But once we reach menopause, with decreasing estrogen levels, muscle loss speeds up. At the same time, bone density can drop by up to 20% in the first five to seven years after menopause. It sounds grim, but here's the twist. Without enough weight-bearing and resistance exercise, the body begins quietly dismantling its own scaffolding. Our muscles, bones, and strength we once took for granted when we were younger. When I first learned this, it became my strongest motivator to prioritize lifting weights two or three times a week

Strength training sends a clear message to your body: "We still need you! Stay strong."

It's about maintaining muscle, safeguarding bone density, enhancing balance (goodbye, unexpected wobbles), and boosting your energy and resilience; not just to get through midlife, but to thrive during it and well beyond.

One of the biggest misconceptions I hear from women is: "I don't want to lift weights; I don't want to bulk up." Let's clear that up right now. Women don't naturally bulk up from lifting weights, and this is even less likely during midlife when estrogen and testosterone levels are lower. Building large, bulky muscles requires high levels of testosterone and specific intensive training, like what bodybuilders do.

What strength training does is help you tighten soft areas, reshape your body, and feel confident in your skin. And you don't need a gym membership or fancy equipment, just a pair of dumbbells or resistance bands at home can be highly effective.

Benefits Strength Training

During menopause, strength training becomes even more crucial as it actively helps keep your bones healthy. Every time you lift, push, or pull against resistance, you place beneficial stress on your bones. This encourages them to absorb calcium and minerals needed to rebuild and strengthen.

This natural process, called bone remodeling, becomes especially important as estrogen levels drop. Research shows that lifting heavy weights not only signals your bones to rebuild but may also activate estrogen receptors in the bone itself. This gives your body extra support at a time when natural protection is declining.

But the benefits go far beyond your bone health. Muscle tissue is metabolically active, meaning it continues to work even while you're at rest. Just one pound of muscle burns about six to ten calories each day, compared to only two to three calories burned by fat tissue. It may sound small, but those numbers add up. Building and maintaining muscle through strength training creates a more efficient internal engine. It helps regulate blood sugar, manage weight, and improve your overall metabolic health.

How to Strength Train

There's no single perfect method. What matters most is finding a style that fits your body, energy, and schedule. Strength training exercises can be performed with different equipment or just your body weight. Examples include:

- Bodyweight Exercises. Squats, lunges, push-ups, planks, and glute bridges. Ideal for at home or holiday workouts.

- Dumbbells and Resistance Bands. Bicep curls, bent-over rows, overhead presses, and weighted squats.

- Weight Machines. Great for beginners to guide movement safely and typically target one muscle group at a time.

- Cable Machines. Enable full-body, functional movements, perfect for weighted pulls, pushes, lunges, and squats. One of my personal favorites for a total-body workout.

- Pilates. Reformer or mat-based exercises for low-impact strength training.

For those with experience and a level of control and fitness:

- Kettlebell Workouts. Dynamic and great for functional strength.

- TRX Suspension Training. Excellent for stability, core, and functional strength.

- Functional Movement Drills. Combining strength and cardio in real-life movement patterns.

When it comes to strength training, remember to start gently and don't overdo it, especially when you're just starting out. A little next-day muscle ache is normal, but you shouldn't be in so much pain that even sitting down on the toilet feels like an Olympic event. That kind of "no pain, no gain" mindset might have worked in your twenties but, at midlife, it's wiser to aim for a gentle reminder that you've worked out, not the kind of discomfort that makes you plot your bathroom trips. The goal is consistency, not punishment.

Different Types of Strength Training

Bodyweight Strength Training

This is the ideal starting point if you're new to exercise or want something gentle and easy to do. Bodyweight exercises help build basic strength, improve joint movement, and reconnect you with your body's natural movement patterns. And don't underestimate their impact. When done regularly, these simple movements tone and strengthen your entire body.

Bodyweight training uses your own body as resistance. Think squats, lunges, push-ups, planks, wall sits, and glute bridges. No equipment needed, just you and some space to move.

Try 2 to 3 sessions each week, starting with 15 to 20 minutes per session. Begin with two rounds and choose five simple exercises such as squats, knee push-ups, glute bridges, wall sits, and bird dogs. Rest for about a minute between rounds, or until your breathing feels steady again. Focus on slow, controlled movements and good form. Aim for 10 to 12 repetitions per exercise, or as many as you can do well, because quality matters more than quantity.

If you're new to strength training, it's worth investing in a few sessions with a personal trainer. Learning proper form early on helps you get the most out of each move and protects you from injury.

Dumbbells and Resistance Bands

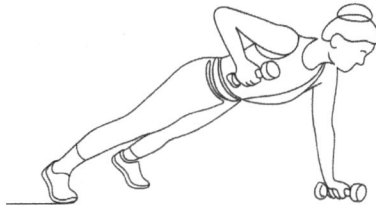

Adding light resistance with dumbbells or resistance bands is a great way to enhance your strength training. These simple tools can work all major muscle groups: arms, shoulders, legs, glutes, back, and core.

Start with light to moderate weights, just enough that the last few reps of each exercise feel challenging but manageable. Exercises like bicep curls, bent-over rows, overhead presses, weighted squats, and deadlifts (done with good form) are simple yet highly effective. Resistance bands are also excellent for joint-friendly strength work and travel routines. They're light, portable, and can make even simple moves feel surprisingly effective.

Aim for 2 to 4 workouts per week, alternating between upper-body and lower-body exercises or performing full-body routines. Each session can last from 20 to 40 minutes, depending on your schedule and energy level. This type of strength training tones your body, boosts your metabolism, and creates the sculpted feeling many women desire, all from the comfort of your own home.

Strength Circuits

Short on time? Try strength circuits. They combine several exercises performed one after another with minimal rest. You'll raise your heart rate while building strength, making it a quick and energizing option for busy weeks.

A basic circuit might include five or six exercises, such as squats, lunges, rows, push-ups, shoulder presses, and planks, each performed for 30 to 45 seconds with 15 to 30 seconds of rest between exercises, and a longer break of 1 to 2 minutes at the end of each round. Repeat the circuit two to three times. You can combine body weight and dumbbell moves or even add resistance band for variety and challenge.

Perform circuits two to three times a week for 20 to 30 minutes. They boost endurance, support muscle tone, and keep you feeling strong rather than exhausted.

Weight Machines

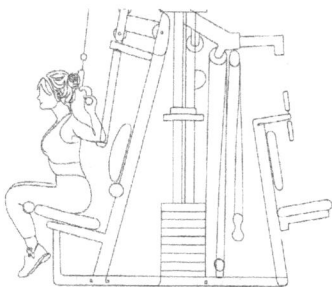

At the gym, you might start with weight machines. They guide your movement and are ideal for beginners. If you want more flexibility and challenge, try cable machines. These allow full-body, functional movements that engage multiple muscle groups. Don't forget about other machines; they're beginner-friendly and gentle on your joints. You can set the range of motion and isolate one muscle group at a time, helping you build strength while protecting your joints along the way.

Try two to three sessions a week, starting with 15-to-20-minute sessions each. Begin with two rounds of five exercises (for example, knee extensions, bench press, biceps curls, leg press, and lat pulldown), resting between rounds. Focus on slow, controlled movement and good form. Don't rush. Aim for a rhythm of three seconds in, hold for one, and three seconds out. This gives your muscles the benefit of "time under tension," which is where real strength is built.

Some gyms offer a free session with a trainer to show you how the machines work. If not, there should be someone on duty who can help. Don't be afraid to ask for help; everyone starts somewhere.

Benefits at a Glance

Here's why resistance training becomes essential in midlife if you want to stay strong, stable, and energized for years to come:

- It safeguards and develops lean muscle. As we age and our hormones change, we naturally lose muscle mass, a condition called sarcopenia. This muscle loss can make us feel weaker, more tired, and less stable on our feet. Strength training helps preserve and even rebuild muscle, which is essential for staying mobile, toned, and resilient.

- It supports your metabolism. Muscle burns more energy than fat, even at rest. Lifting weights helps your body burn calories all day, not just during workouts. This can help prevent the weight gain many women face in midlife.

- It enhances insulin sensitivity. Midlife is often when blood sugar regulation begins to change, making weight gain (especially around the waist) more common. Resistance training helps your muscles absorb glucose more effectively, reducing insulin resistance and stabilizing energy levels.

- It strengthens bones. As estrogen declines, bone loss speeds up, raising the risk of fractures and osteoporosis. But here's the good news: Bones respond to stress. Lifting weights (even light ones) tells your bones to stay strong, dense, and functional. Strength training is one of the most powerful tools for lifelong bone health.

- It boosts confidence, mobility, and strength. Feeling strong in your body changes everything. It's the difference between struggling with groceries and carrying them with ease or watching from the sidelines and joining in with your grandkids. Resistance training restores physical confidence. It also supports balance, posture, and coordination, which are the quiet foundations of aging well and maintaining independence.

How Often and When

Aiming for two to four strength training sessions each week is ideal during menopause. Even 20 to 30 minutes of focused resistance work at home or wherever you are can make a real difference. Sure, your workouts should challenge you, but they shouldn't leave you completely wiped out. The aim is to finish feeling stronger, more energized, and glad you showed up. Not like you need a nap or an ice pack just to recover. And while a little muscle ache is normal, you don't want to be so sore from squats that even sitting down feels like an Olympic event. Think of it as building a gradual build. Add more time and intensity as your strength and confidence grow.

Give yourself at least 48 hours between workouts for proper recovery. Your muscles need that time to repair, rebuild, and grow stronger. Strength training creates tiny micro-tears in your muscle fibers, and it's during rest that your body repairs these fibers, making them more resilient. Skipping recovery can backfire, leading to fatigue, soreness, and even slowing down your progress.

Other key points to remember include:

- Start with light weights. If you're new to strength training, begin with bodyweight exercises or light resistance. Strength training is about progression. That means consistently showing up, listening to your body, and building your foundation one session at a time.

- Focus on form. Quality of movement matters more than quantity. Make sure you perform the exercises safely and effectively. Start where you are, not where you think you should be.

- Incorporate variety. Use a mix of bodyweight, free weights, and resistance bands for balanced strength development.

- Injury prevention. If you're new or unsure where to start, I strongly suggest working with a certified trainer, even if only for a few sessions. They'll teach you proper technique, guide your pace, and help you move safely and confidently.

Take Katherine, for example. Her story is an inspiring reminder of what's possible. After just six months of consistent strength training twice a week, she went from avoiding physical activity to reaching her goals. She can now do full push-ups, garden all day without the back pain that used to hold her back. She even started helping her teenage son with the heavy yard work she once dreaded. But the real goosebump moment? Her follow-up bone density scan was so significant that even her doctor was surprised. Katherine didn't just feel stronger; she was stronger, inside and out.

Finding What Works in Midlife

This was a fascinating discovery during one of my lowest energy phases, when menopause symptoms and chronic fatigue left me depleted. I knew I needed to move, but my old routines, full-body compound exercises, fast-paced circuits, and long power walks only wiped me out. Still, I was determined to find a way to support my body without draining it. That's when I began experimenting.

I realized I could still strength train, but I had to approach it differently. If I sat or lay down and focused on one muscle group at a time, I could lift without overwhelming my system. The moment I tried to combine too many movements at the same time, like squats with overhead presses, I'd finish the workout feeling more drained instead of strong. I let my body set the pace, not a rulebook.

I also swapped long, exhausting cardio treks for gentle ten-to-twenty-minute strolls. If I had more energy, I went farther. If not, I gave myself permission to slow down. Walking in beautiful places—the bush, the beach, quiet parks—became medicine for my nervous system. Soaking in the calm of the natural world felt like a reset for my soul.

Building Strength for the Future

It wasn't about pushing harder anymore. It was about listening, adapting, and choosing what truly supported my body, mind, and mood. Gradually, I began to feel stronger. More grounded. More like me. The change wasn't flashy. It wasn't extreme. Still, it was real and sustainable.

Remember, strength training during menopause is about building a body that supports you for decades to come. A strong, resilient body that carries you through life's seasons with energy, confidence, and grace. Start slowly. Progress gradually. Celebrate the small wins. Because every rep, every intentional move, is a quiet investment in your future self that says, "I'm worth taking care of."

Most of all, trust that this phase of your life is about reinvention. Strength training teaches you to meet yourself where you are, show up, and stay consistent, even if the world feels uncertain. When your body feels strong, your mind feels steadier. Your energy becomes clearer. And life feels just a little more doable.

Focusing on age-proofing your body and feeling capable in your second act, include functional, core, and postural training that improve your range of motion and flexibility.

Below, I've outlined some of the most effective ways to move with purpose and build lasting strength from the inside out.

Functional Movements

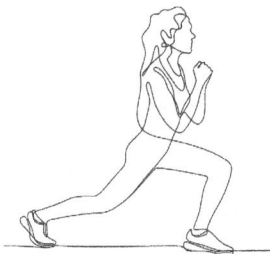

Functional training mimics real-life movements, such as lifting, squatting, rotating, stepping, and carrying. Think of lifting your dog into the car, carrying a heavy laundry basket, or pulling a suitcase through the airport. These are all functional movements. When performed intentionally, they also serve as strength training exercises. It's about staying strong for life, not just for the gym.

Examples include squats, push-ups (on knees or against a wall to make them easier), glute bridges, step-ups, and any exercises that strengthen your core, especially those involving twisting motions. These moves help with everyday tasks such as climbing stairs, lifting groceries from your car, or picking up shoes off the floor.

You can also incorporate functional strength exercises, such as step-ups, kettlebell deadlifts, or loaded carries, into your weekly routine. Even 10 to 15 minutes a couple of times a week, can make a noticeable difference.

Let your breath guide your movement. Breathing deeply while you move helps regulate your nervous system and keeps you present. If your breath becomes strained or you feel short of breath, pause and come back when you're ready.

Enhancing Balance

This is one of the most underrated yet essential forms of training at midlife. As estrogen declines, coordination and stability naturally weaken, which increases the risk of falls and injuries. Simple daily practices make a difference. Try standing on one leg while brushing your teeth or waiting for the kettle to boil. These small actions engage multiple muscle groups, your core, glutes, and legs, and strengthen the small stabilizers in your hips and ankles. Pilates is a wonderful way to build balance and body awareness while gently strengthening your whole system.

Start by standing on one leg for 30 seconds, then work up to a full minute. Once you've mastered that, try closing your eyes. You'll be surprised at how much more your balance and focus are challenged. Over time, this practice improves posture, joint health, and overall confidence in daily movement. Walking backward offers another surprising way to challenge your muscles and coordination. Research shows it improves knee strength, sharpens cognitive function, and enhance balance. And then there's tai chi, often called "meditation in motion" - a beautiful, mindful way to connect body, breath, and balance.

Postural Support, Core Work, and Mobility

Have you ever noticed how older people seem to shrink? Shoulders round forward, the head tilts down, and steps turn into shuffles. Devices and aches often make this more pronounced, but one of the earliest signs of aging is poor posture. That's why posture deserves special attention at midlife. The way you stand, walk, and carry yourself doesn't just affect how you look; it influences your energy, confidence, and mobility in the decades to come.

As you start increasing your activity and intensity, you may notice stiffer joints, or you may struggle to get into a deep squat position. This is no reason to stop. Instead, see it as a signal from your body to give it more care. Decades of postural habits will become more pronounced now, without the buffering effects of estrogen on your joints, connective tissue, and muscles. So, why not take the hint and fine-tune your posture and range of motion? Incorporating some core and mobility exercises can make a remarkable difference. Strengthening your postural muscles and improving your joint mobility can even create a more streamlined, lean look (hello Pilates-physique).

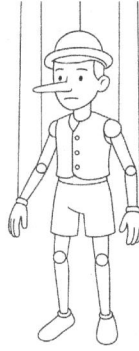

I often describe posture as walking upright from the top of your head, like a "Pinocchio puppet." Imagine a string gently pulling you taller, with your arms and legs moving gracefully at your sides. It's simple but transformative to picture it this way. Practice it consciously, and you may find yourself looking five inches taller and ten years younger.

Whether your goal is to move more freely or to tighten your inner corset, postural and stretching workouts such as Pilates and yoga have multiple benefits. They are accessible and can be scaled up easily, and you'll get instant results in the way you feel. They have several of the other benefits of exercise, such as mood-boosting qualities, joint health, cardiovascular health, social connection, and greater mindfulness.

If heading to a studio is too daunting, check out YouTube or apps like YogaGlo for some popular accounts. Many teachers offer free sessions and have a large library of 10-to-60-minute videos available online. Having a schedule or small subscription helps you stay accountable and build consistency.

For more personalized results, try reformer Pilates, yoga therapy, or guided sessions with a physiotherapist or trainer. Targeted programs help correct long-held imbalances like tight hip flexors, rounded shoulders, or a dominant side. Do not hesitate to ask for at-home exercises, because you will change patterns faster with consistent practice woven into daily life.

Even 45 minutes a week of posture-focused movement lowers your risk of falls, eases back or hip pain, and reduces tension headaches. If you are already active, two to three sessions of 30 to 60 minutes will enhance strength and mobility without taxing your body. Done well, this kind of training leaves you standing taller, moving more freely, and feeling energized long after you step off the mat.

Pilates for Your Core

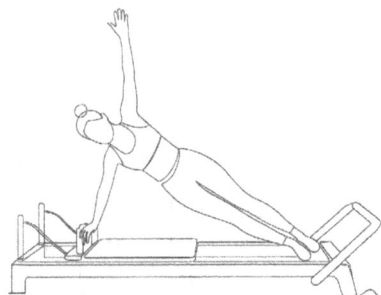

If you prefer more structure and mindfulness, Pilates (especially on the reformer) is ideal. Pilates offers low-impact strength training that supports posture, core control, and joint health. It is beginner-friendly, as the machine helps you stay aligned while allowing easy modifications depending on your energy. The different spring strengths build resistance in surprising ways. Less resistance often means more control, as your deep stabilizers work harder. Most classes last 45 to 50 minutes, but if you are new, start with a private session to learn the basics and build confidence. Aim for one to two sessions a week and avoid high-intensity versions. The goal is strength and resilience, not exhaustion.

Think of your body in menopause as a team that has lost a few key players. Coordination, balance, and core strength can all take a hit. Pilates brings everything back into alignment, improving stability, and reminding your body how to move with grace again. As estrogen dips, your spine, pelvic floor, and deep core can weaken, leaving you feeling stiff or unsteady. Pilates strengthens these areas and helps restore both confidence and connection.

Two-time World Cup Champion Megan Rapinoe put it perfectly: "Pilates strengthens from the inside out." It does not just tone your abs; it rebuilds your foundation. Hormonal changes in midlife affect spinal flexibility, muscle tone, bone density, and posture. Pilates helps protect both spinal mobility and bone density while it works the glutes, back, core, and pelvic floor to support posture and balance.

By consciously engaging your pelvic floor during movements, you strengthen not only the muscles that support continence and pelvic stability and improve overall core function. Breathing, activating, and releasing the pelvic floor creates a resilient base that supports every other move you make.

For women with back pain, pelvic instability, or joint issues, Pilates is especially life-changing. The mindful breathwork also calms the nervous system, an often-overlooked part of midlife wellbeing.

When I was deep in back pain and stiffness, Pilates became my way back. I did not just get stronger; I reconnected with myself. I stood taller, moved more freely, and felt confident in my body again. I see the same with my clients. They arrive stiff or unsure. Then, within weeks, they say they feel stronger, taller, steadier, and more at ease. That is the beauty of Pilates. The results are both immediate and lasting.

One of its greatest gifts is adaptability. Some days, you may want the challenge of reformer work. On other days, you may crave gentle mat practice, breathwork, or stretching. Both count as wins. If you are new, begin slowly with a few private sessions. Learn the form, build your base, and give yourself time to adjust.

Pilates is more than a strength and core workout. It is a reset, a breathing practice, and a stabilizing anchor in this season of change.

Yoga for Strength and Balance

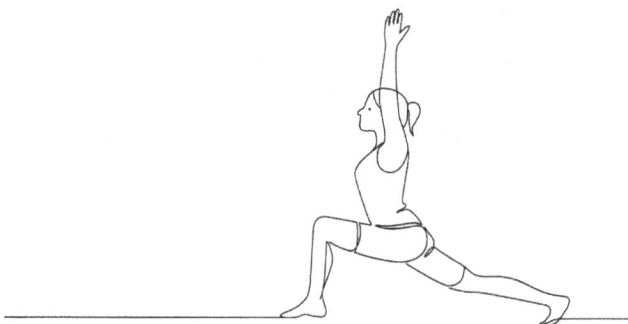

Perhaps you've never considered yoga before, or maybe you tried but didn't like it. The good news? Just like strength training or Pilates, yoga is incredibly versatile and adaptable. One of the biggest gifts in midlife is that listening to your body is built into the practice. This means you're far less likely to push beyond your changing limits because awareness, not force, is the focus.

The most common objection I hear from people new to yoga is that they "aren't flexible," which is, of course, no prerequisite. Most forms of yoga are designed to help you get more flexible while also building balance, strength and mobility. Dynamic styles like Power Yoga and Bikram include standing sequences, balances, and weight-bearing postures that not only improve flexibility but also help maintain bone strength and lean muscle, both vital in midlife.

Practicing in a heated room can further challenge your cardiovascular system and support temperature regulation, but be sure to stay well hydrated. In my thirties, I was hooked on Bikram yoga. I thrived on those thirty-day challenges in the heat, pushing myself to stay the course. But when perimenopause arrived, the intensity that once energized me started to leave me completely wiped out. That shift was my lesson: Yoga can evolve with you. From vigorous flows that build stamina to gentler practices, like supportive yin and restorative yoga, that soothe the nervous system and improve mobility, there's a style for every season.

If the spiritual side of yoga isn't your thing, choose teachers who keep cues practical and focus on physical alignment and breath. Yoga can be as grounded or as soulful as you wish, it's about what serves you best right now. If you are interested in fostering a better mind-body connection, achieving stress relief, enhancing mobility, and improving your posture and sleep simultaneously, finding the type of yoga and instructor that resonates with you is one of the kindest choices you can make for your midlife body.

If you're most interested in yoga for nervous system reset and stress relief, read on, as there is a section on this.

Cardiovascular Exercise

Moderate Intensity Cardio

During this phase of life, your body undergoes hormonal shifts that impact cortisol, insulin, joints, muscles, and your ability to recover (you name it, really!). Long, steady-state cardio sessions, like running, cycling, or walking at the same pace for an hour or more, may no longer deliver that endorphin high and can instead leave you feeling flat or wiped out. With less estrogen, cortisol stays elevated longer, slows down recovery and promotes fat storage, particularly around the midsection.

At the same time, muscle preservation and blood sugar regulation become trickier. Long bouts of cardio, especially without proper fueling, can lead to muscle breakdown and increase insulin resistance, leaving you tired, hungry, and frustrated by stubborn weight gain.

So, if your usual cardio routine now leaves you feeling anxious, puffy, or simply run down. Listen to your feedback system! Your body isn't broken. It's asking for a new kind of partnership for your sessions.

Research suggests, shorter, focused sessions -around 20 to 30 minutes of moderate to high-intensity intervals. This can help manage weight, support insulin sensitivity, and boost mood.

That said, where you start matters. If you finish your workouts feeling energized, keep doing what works. But if you're returning to exercise or noticing more fatigue, let your breathing be a good guide. Warm up well, keep intervals short enough to recover within a few breaths and keep total sessions at a length that feels sustainable.

For most of us, that will mean low to moderate intensity of steady-state cardio (where you maintain the intensity at a relatively constant level) is okay for up to an hour, or even longer, if you are fairly fit.

For interval sessions, start with 10 minutes and build to 30 minutes as your endurance improves. Beginners might do 15 to 30 seconds of higher intensity followed by a minute or more of recovery; fitter women might extend bursts to 60 seconds with 30 to 60 seconds of rest.

Beware the endorphin trap: that post-workout high can mask fatigue and make it easy to overdo it. If you're struggling to recover or feel wired after class, that's your sign to pull back. You can still challenge yourself, just don't chase exhaustion. A good example? Skip the spin class with blaring music and "go harder!" commands. Those external cues drown out your body's signals. The real goal is vitality, not burnout.

The benefits of cardio on weight loss and overall health can be a big plus, so cardio is still an arrow in your quiver. About 150 minutes a week, spread over four to five days, (if you're moderately fit) of low to moderate intensity cardio can age-proof your cardiovascular system and lower stress levels. Golf, tennis, brisk walking, swimming, and running all count as physical activity.

As your joints and body also need a bit more love to prevent injuries, you just want to make sure you also include postural work, range of motion, and strength training.

Cardio's Benefits

Smart cardio does far more than just burning calories. It supports your body from the inside out.

Here's how:

- Manages insulin sensitivity and blood sugar balance. As estrogen levels decline, your cells can become more resistant to insulin, making weight gain, especially around the middle, more likely. Regular, moderate cardio helps your body use insulin more effectively, reducing blood sugar spikes and supporting a steadier metabolism.

- Improves sleep and lifts your mood. Gentle to moderate movement releases feel-good neurotransmitters, like serotonin and dopamine. It eases anxiety, irritability, and emotional swings, and helps regulate your circadian rhythm, for deeper, more restful sleep, especially when done earlier in the day.

- Strengthens bones and heart. Cardio keeps your heart healthy, supports circulation, and helps maintain healthy blood pressure and cholesterol levels. Weight-bearing activities, such as walking and hiking, help strengthen bones, reducing the risk of osteoporosis.

- Sharpens focus and cools hot flashes. Regular movement boosts blood flow to the brain, helping clear brain fog, and sharpens concentration. It can also help regulate body temperature and intensity of hot flashes.

Best Midlife Cardio

The best kind of cardio at this stage of life is the kind that works *with* your hormones, not against them. Think low-impact, joint-friendly movement that feels good, supports your energy, and builds strength without leaving you exhausted. The goal isn't to go harder, but to move consistently in ways that build you up.

Here are some great low-impact options:

- Brisk Walking. 20 to 60 minutes, three to five times per week. One of the simplest and most effective forms of cardio. Walking improves heart health, supports lymphatic flow, and helps regulate blood sugar, all while being gentle on the joints. Bonus: walking outdoors also lowers cortisol and boosts mood and reconnects you with nature.

- Gentle Hikes. Once to twice a week. Adding hills and uneven terrain builds strength, balance, and coordination. Hiking also doubles as a mental reset, combining fresh air and natural scenery that soothes stress and enhances mental clarity.

- Swimming. 20 to 30 minutes, one to three times per week. The ultimate joint-friendly workout. Swimming strengthens heart and lung health, tones the body without stressing the joints, and keeps you cool (especially helpful if you're managing hot flashes). It also encourages deep breathing, which supports your nervous system.

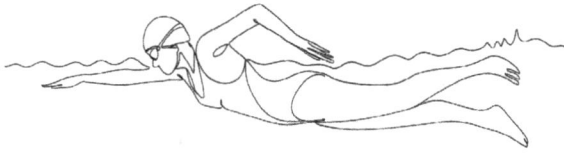

- Cycling. 20 to 45 minutes, one to three times per week. Whether it's a gentle spin on a stationary bike or a casual ride through the park, cycling boosts lower-body strength and circulation with minimal impact on knees and hips. It's also a mood-lifter and great for endorphins.

- HIIT. Start with a 5-minute warm-up and finish with a 5-minute cool-down. Try short bursts of effort, such as 30 seconds of faster cycling, walking, or hill climbs, followed by one to two minutes at a slow pace to recover. Repeat this pattern for 10 to 30 minutes. A few rounds, once or twice a week, are enough to fire up your metabolism and support insulin sensitivity without hijacking your nervous system.

- Dancing. Ten to 30 minutes, as often as it brings you joy! Dancing boosts coordination, balance, mood, and heart health. It also reconnects you with your creativity and emotional expression. Whether it's a class or a solo kitchen dance party, it counts.

- Recreational Sports. One to two times per week. These are wonderful social forms of movement. Tennis adds agility and quick bursts of energy. Golf encourages walking, focus and precision. Both offer community, fresh air, and challenge, all of which are beneficial for a thriving mind and body.

Variety Builds Strength

Many of us stick to what we know. Same walk. Same class. Same routine. It feels safe and familiar. But over time, your body adjusts. Progress slows, and motivation fades.

A little change can make a big difference. Try new moves. Adjust your reps. Lift a bit heavier. Change your pace. Even small tweaks wake up your muscles and mind.

It can be as simple as swapping squats for step-ups. Replacing a walking route with a few quick bursts of hill climbing. Variety keeps things fresh and helps you keep improving. Movement should change as you do.

Mix it up. Your body will respond, and your mind will stay engaged.

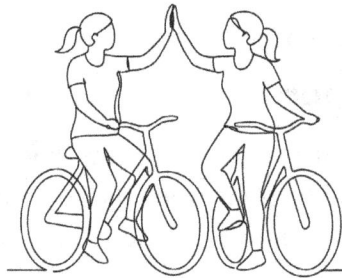

Reset Your Metabolism

Let's talk about something many women in midlife feel but don't always know how to fix. The slow, sluggish metabolism that seems to hit out of nowhere. You're moving your body, maybe even eating better than ever, but that stubborn belly fat or lower-body weight just won't budge.

You can turn things around with the right kind of strength training. Science shows that compound movements, exercises that use multiple big muscle groups at once, create a strong hormonal response that boosts metabolism for up to 48 hours after your session is done. That's right; your body continues to burn energy long after you've rolled up your mat.

These types of workouts also boost key hormones, like human growth hormone and testosterone. They help you burn fat, build muscle tone, improve mood, and that subtle yet powerful feeling of vitality that often disappears during this stage of life.

You don't need long, punishing sessions. You can complete these short, targeted workouts at home in 20 to 30 minutes, using just a pair of dumbbells or your body weight. Try simple, compound exercises such as squats with bicep curls, lunges with shoulder presses, deadlifts with upright rows, or step-ups with side raises. These targeted workouts create metabolic stress, which simply means your body works harder to recover. That extra effort helps burn stubborn fat that won't go away with cardio alone.

What makes this even more exciting is how they'll make you feel. These types of workouts help sharpen your mind, improve blood sugar regulation, stabilize your mood, and naturally boost your energy. You'll begin to feel stronger, clearer, and more in control. Strength training doesn't just change your body. It brings back your spark.

Matching Movement to Hormonal Rhythms

As estrogen naturally declines, your body reacts differently to exercise. This signals that your body is adjusting, prompting you to modify how and when you move. Suddenly, timing becomes crucial.

Consider my client Sarah as an example. She'd been dedicated to her five a.m. spin classes for years. But now, they were leaving her completely wiped out. Her sleep suffered, energy crashed in the mid-afternoon, and she couldn't understand why. The problem wasn't effort. It was timing.

Early mornings are when cortisol naturally peaks. Adding intense exercise on top of that was overloading her already stressed system. Once she moved her training to mid-morning, everything improved. She felt energized, recovered more quickly, and no longer needed to crawl into bed before sunset.

Here's how aligning movement with your natural rhythm helps:

- Early morning. Ideal for gentle, grounding movement, like stretching, breath-led Pilates, or a light walk. Cortisol is already high, so avoid further spiking it with tough workout sessions.

- Mid-morning to early afternoon. This is your power window. Body temperature, coordination, and strength peak here. It's an excellent time for strength training, moderate circuits, or focused Pilates.

- Late afternoon. Your pain tolerance and endurance rise naturally, making this an excellent time for moderate cardio, like cycling, brisk walking, or swimming.

- Evenings. Begin to wind down with mobility work, gentle yoga, or restorative stretching to prep your body (and nervous system) for quality sleep.

If you finish a workout feeling wired but drained, can't sleep, or crave sugar, you're pushing too hard. Recovery matters most now. Create your own energy map. Notice when you feel strong or tired. Pay attention to how different workouts affect your mood and sleep. As hormones shift, so will your energy. Be flexible. On low-energy days, choose gentle movement. On higher-energy days, lift heavy weights or move with purpose.

When you move in harmony with your body instead of fighting against it, you access deeper strength, clearer thinking, and more lasting vitality.

Making Movement Fit Your Life

Movement doesn't have to happen in a gym or in fancy workout gear to count. As a trainer, I've heard every excuse: "I don't have enough time," "I'm too sore," "I'm too tired," "I can't afford it." But the truth is, once you understand how vital movement is, you realize you can't afford not to move. It shapes your energy, strength, and confidence. You stop putting it behind Netflix binges or extra sleep-ins.

I've learned to weave movement into my life wherever I go. Some of my favorite workouts have happened outside the studio. When traveling, I've often had to get creative. On a recent trip to visit my brother in the UK, I took my teenage nephews to a park in central London. Sunshine, open space, and a few outdoor weight machines were all we needed. With some encouragement from their cheeky auntie, we laughed our way through push-ups, sit-ups, and sprints. That playful competition made exercise fun and simple.

Even when staying for weeks on a boat, I found ways to keep my body moving. I packed kettlebells and a rebounder, bouncing every morning on the deck while lifting weights, heart pumping and spirits high. At sunrise and sunset, I'd paddleboard with my little Aussie terrier Baxter perched on the front of the board, or dive in for a swim around the boat, a family tradition to do before lunch. Whenever I could, activity became part of my daily habits.

My clients do the same. Lynne, who travels constantly for work, trains with me via Zoom session in tiny hotel rooms. We've created 50-minute routines using nothing but bodyweight with enough to stretch, strengthen, and keep her energized.

The most important thing is finding something you love and doing it consistently. As we've already talked about, muscles atrophy as we age. Without movement, we lose strength, mobility, and confidence far too quickly. But with it, we keep our bodies supple, our minds sharp, and our spirit lifted. Movement truly heals.

The truth is, I see it in my clients all the time. Unless they hit a crisis point, many don't prioritize movement. But the ones who do? Magic happens. They stand taller, move with more ease, radiate energy, and often transform their lives completely with confidence.

So, start today, one small step at a time. Call a friend and walk instead of meeting for a drink. Stretch for ten minutes before bed. Park the car a little farther away and walk to work. Try a new sport, maybe golf. Be the best you can be. It's up to you to make a difference in your life.

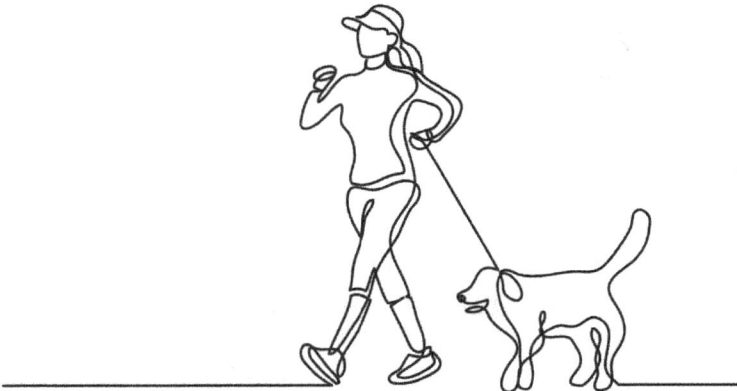

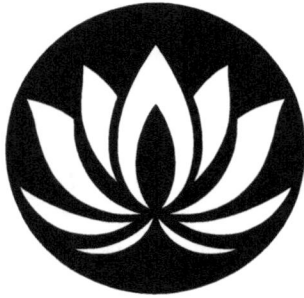

Pillar Four –
Rest and Recovery

"Growing into your future with health and grace and beauty doesn't have to take all your time. It rather requires a dedication to caring for yourself as if you were rare and precious, which you are, and regarding all life around you as equally so, which it is."

– VICTORIA MORAN, AUTHOR

In the chaos of midlife, it's easy to forget that you are rare and precious. But as Victoria Moran so beautifully reminds us, this chapter of life doesn't require you to do more, it asks you to care more deeply. Not out of pressure, but out of reverence. Because, during menopause, caring for yourself with tenderness isn't a luxury, it's a lifeline.

Between hormonal rollercoasters, the unrelenting pressure to hold everything together, and the ever-present hum of stress, sleep often becomes a casualty. It starts slipping through your fingers like sand, leaving you exhausted, edgy, and wondering why you're wide awake at three a.m., replaying conversations from 2007.

That constant hum of tension? That's your nervous system, on high alert, overstimulated by cortisol spikes, disrupted rhythms, and a brain that refuses to switch off. And it's no wonder. Menopause puts your nervous system in the crosshairs: estrogen dips, melatonin dwindles, and stress hormones start throwing midnight raves. You're not broken, you're simply being asked to support yourself differently.

CHAPTER 14

Active Recovery

"Do something today that your future self will

thank you for."

–SEAN PATRICK FLANERY

Movement and Recovery

Recovery at midlife becomes a fully strategic yet intuitive lifestyle. It involves eating enough protein to repair and rebuild, prioritizing sleep that truly restores, staying well-hydrated, fueling your body before and after exercise, and perhaps most importantly, learning to manage stress instead of masking it with coffee.

Take Michelle, one of my powerhouse clients. As a former athlete, she was used to pushing hard, wearing fatigue like a badge of honor. But during menopause, that approach left her sore for days and drained of energy. We swapped the "grind harder" mindset for a balanced routine: strength training a few times a week, restorative movement, and gentle cardio. The result? Her energy returned, her strength rebuilt, and she stopped burning out.

This is the beauty of energy-smart exercise: It respects your body's rhythms. It's not about proving anything; it's building something strong and sustainable. Movement now becomes a gift, calming anxiety, protecting bones, balancing hormones, and helping you feel at home in your body again.

So, instead of chasing exhaustion, choose workouts that leave you feeling replenished. That could be weight training, yoga, Pilates, hiking, swimming, or dancing in your kitchen. What matters most isn't the *what*, but the *how*: how it makes you feel. And often, doing it with others adds joy and consistency, whether it's laughing through squats or walking with a friend.

It may surprise you to know: Your body doesn't rebuild during the workout. It rebuilds during rest. That's when muscles repair, hormones recalibrate, and your nervous system resets. Two to three strength sessions a week, paired with restorative practices and deep rest, will do more for your metabolism, mood, and mobility than any boot camp schedule.

Stillness isn't weakness; it's medicine. Recovery is where your next level of strength is waiting.

The Importance of Rest and Recovery

Recovery done right is a strategic and intelligent move. It's also deeply healing. When you begin to honor the rhythm of exertion and rest, you step out of the hustle loop and into a state of long-term strength, energy, and nervous system balance.

At midlife, when fatigue, sleep struggles, or stress may hit harder, rest becomes your greatest ally. Gentle tools like meditation, breathwork, journaling, massage, or acupuncture help reset the system and bring you back into balance. Without them, the body risks staying stuck in overdrive, leaving you inflamed, drained, and discouraged.

I've learned this lesson personally. Every time I tried to push through fatigue, I paid for it later with deeper crashes. Now I guard recovery like I do any workout. It's non-negotiable. Some days, that looks like an Epsom salt bath, a massage, or simply allowing a slow morning without rushing.

If you've been feeling guilty about slowing down, release it. Rest is not weakness. Stillness is medicine. Recovery is where your next chapter of strength begins.

Active Recovery

Not all movement has to be about intensity or breaking a sweat. Some of the most nourishing practices are the ones that restore rather than deplete, the kind that give back more energy than they use. At midlife, when your nervous system, joints, and hormones are calling for more care, these forms of movement become medicine.

A slow walk under the trees, a gentle Pilates flow, or rolling out your mat for restorative yoga can calm your stress response, boost circulation, and ease tension in ways a high-intensity workout never could. This isn't doing less; it's moving smarter. Choosing activities that replenish your reserves, soften your edges, and remind your body that strength can be nurtured as well as built.

Yoga and Tai Chi

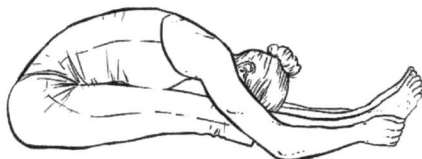

Yin and Restorative Yoga

One of the most beneficial restorative styles during this menopausal phase is yin yoga. Unlike fast-paced flows that might leave you gasping for your forgotten youth, yin is slow, restorative, and focuses on long, passive holds, typically lasting three to five minutes. These holds allow the body to release deeply held tension from the fascia and joints.

Yin is deeply soothing for the nervous system, gently guiding you into a state of rest. The slow, steady breathing practiced in yin stimulates the vagus nerve, your body's natural "calm switch," helping to reduce stress, lower the heart rate, and bring you back into balance. This combination of breath, stillness, and mindful awareness also supports hormone regulation, reduces inflammation, eases fatigue, and encourages the natural release of melatonin, promoting deeper, more restorative sleep.

In a yin class, the instructor gently guides you into poses that are held for several minutes. Some, like the dragon poses, will test your patience and your edges. Yet it is in that stillness that the release comes. By the end of class, I would often feel unspooled and lighter, as though the twists and long holds had wrung out all the tension I had been carrying inside. Yin became less about powering through and more about unwinding, creating space for calm to settle in.

But yin isn't the only style with benefits in midlife. Restorative yoga takes this softness even further, using props like bolsters, blankets, and blocks to fully support your body so you can drop into complete relaxation without effort. It is like being gently cradled into stillness, allowing stress hormones to settle and the nervous system to downshift. Gentle hatha yoga, on the other hand, offers simple postures with mindful breathing; it's accessible, grounding, and perfect for reconnecting with your body on days when energy feels low, but you still crave movement.

Together, these slower styles remind you that yoga doesn't always have to be about bending yourself into a pretzel or powering through sweat-drenched sequences. At midlife, yoga can be a sanctuary. It's soothing, supportive, and profoundly aligned with what your changing body and spirit truly need.

Tai Chi

And then there's the gentle practice of Tai Chi, often called "meditation in motion." With its slow, flowing movements, coordinated breathing, and mindful intention, Tai Chi provides an incredibly gentle yet effective way to support the body and mind during menopause. Originally developed as a martial art, Tai Chi enhances balance, coordination, posture, and mental clarity.

It has been shown to soothe the nervous system, reduce cortisol levels, improve sleep quality, and support heart health. The slow, circular movements also lubricate stiff joints, boost energy flow (what the Chinese call "qi"), and gently build strength without draining your energy. I often weave a few simple Tai Chi moves into the start of my classes to shift energy, ground us, and bring mind and body into sync for the session ahead.

Whether you find yourself melting into a bolster during a Yin Yoga session or drifting through a Tai Chi routine, both practices offer powerful ways to nourish your nervous system, rebuild strength, and reconnect with the incredible wisdom of your changing body. And let's be honest, there's something wonderfully rebellious about choosing stillness and softness when the world keeps yelling, "Do more!"

Modern Forms of Active Recovery

Active recovery doesn't have to be complicated or boring. There are endless ways to move gently while giving your body the chance to restore. Foam rolling can feel surprisingly active (try holding a plank while rolling tight quads), a tennis ball works wonders on stubborn spots like hip flexors, and resistance bands are perfect for simple mobility moves like leg circles or shoulder figure eights. Yoga therapy, like the approach taught by physiotherapist Simon Borg-Olivier, blends breath, mobility, and calm. He describes it beautifully: *"Doing yoga therapy should feel like sitting in a warm bath. You should feel relaxed and calm while moving."*

But sometimes, recovery is less about tools and more about tuning in. When clients arrive at my studio saying they are "fine" but clearly running on fumes, we often switch gears. Instead of pushing through a workout, we shift to what I call "working in" exercises: slow, yin-based movements that rebuild energy instead of draining it. These simple, restorative practices calm the nervous system, boost circulation, and gently bring you back into your body when life feels scattered.

You don't need a whole routine. One or two poses, chosen intuitively, can ground you, soften tension, or spark just enough energy to carry you through the day. The key is listening. Let your breath guide you. Let your body whisper what it needs. Because, in midlife, true strength isn't always about pushing harder; it's about finding your way back to flow.

My Favorite Active Recovery Movements

- Arm Swings (Qigong style). Simple, rhythmic swings that release tension, calm the mind, and boost circulation. Just a few minutes can shift your whole energy.

- Legs Up the Wall. A deeply calming pose that eases anxiety, improves circulation, and helps with swollen legs or sleepless nights.

- Child's Pose. A soothing forward fold that releases the lower back, hips, and mind, and offers a comforting reset when life feels heavy.

- Cat-Cow Stretch. Flowing movement that loosens the spine, gently massages the back and belly to help melt tension away.

- Downward Dog. A full-body reset that stretches, strengthens, and reenergizes. Lengthens tight muscles and resets the spine after sitting or standing too long.

- Sphinx Pose. A gentle backbend that undoes hours of sitting and opens the chest, counteracts slouching, and eases lower back tightness, especially after hours at a desk.

- Bridge Pose. Strengthens the back body and glutes while gently lifting mood and energy.

- Passive Recovery. Sometimes the best reset is no movement at all, just lying down feeling the earth support you, breathing deeply, or soaking in a warm bath. It lowers cortisol, restores hormones, and replenishes energy.

Scheduled Rest Days

Train wisely by building recovery into your plan. Rest days aren't an afterthought; they're as essential as your workouts. The biggest mistake many people make is waiting until they're completely exhausted or sore before hitting pause. By then, your body is already in catch-up mode.

Just as you schedule strength sessions, yoga, or Pilates classes, you should also schedule active recovery sessions and rest. This is when the real transformation happens. Muscles repair, hormones recalibrate, inflammation eases, and your nervous system shifts out of "go-mode." Without this reset, you risk plateauing, burnout, or injury.

Midlife makes this even more important. With fluctuating hormones, your nervous system is already on higher alert, more fragile, more easily tipped into stress mode. Rest days act as a calming signal, reminding your body it's safe to power down. Gentle pauses help regulate cortisol, soothe frazzled nerves, and create the conditions for deeper recovery.

Think of rest as strategic, not slacking. These days allow your body to adapt, recharge, and come back stronger. When you honor recovery, you don't lose momentum; you create the foundation for sustainable strength, steadier energy, and a calmer, more resilient nervous system.

Recovery Support

Over the years, through plenty of trial and error, I've learned to treat my body, nervous system, and mind with deep respect. Prevention really is better than cure, whether through food, movement, lifestyle, or therapies that keep you in balance. For me, that looks like regular massage to release tension, acupuncture to restore energy flow, and the occasional visit to a chiropractor or osteopath to stay aligned and moving freely.

I've built a trusted circle of health professionals I see regularly, and I often share their details with friends and clients. Having that support team is a strategy for prevention rather than cure, not a luxury. Just as you need the right collaborators to run a business, you also need the right people around you to care for your body. Over time, our bodies need *more* support, not less. And when you invest in your body's maintenance and recovery, you're choosing to live with more ease, energy, and longevity.

Think of recovery like seasoning: just enough makes everything work better. Small, intentional practices sprinkled through your week can reduce inflammation, support healing, and keep you feeling strong. If you've pushed hard in a workout or tackled a long hike, balance it with a recovery activity to soften the impact and help your body adapt.

Here are a few examples you can weave into your rest days or even in small bursts throughout the day to accelerate recovery:

Cold Exposure (Ice Baths, Cold Showers, or Ocean Dips)

Cold therapy may feel like the latest wellness trend, but it's been around for thousands of years. The Greeks and Romans swore by cold water for recovery and rejuvenation, and today science is backing up what they already knew: Short, controlled bursts of cold can benefit both body and mind.

Cold exposure helps reduce inflammation, improve circulation, boost energy, and lift mood by triggering endorphins and norepinephrine, your body's natural "feel-good" chemicals. For midlife women, gentle cold therapy can be especially helpful for easing hormone-related inflammation, fatigue, or brain fog. Some research even suggests it may support metabolic health and insulin sensitivity, which often shift during perimenopause and menopause.

If you're curious, start small:

- Contrast showers. End a warm shower with 30 seconds of cold, building up to one or two minutes.

- Ocean or pool dips. A quick plunge can invigorate your system, especially in the morning.

- Ice baths. If trying at home, keep it short (30 seconds to 2 minutes), focus on calm breathing, and always warm up afterward.

The key is to stay mindful. Cold exposure is a hormetic stressor. It can build resilience, but only in balance with rest. If you're already depleted, anxious, or stressed, skip it that day and choose something more nurturing, like a warm bath or restorative yoga.

Athletes often use ice baths or ocean plunges to recover after punishing sessions, but for everyday midlife bodies, less is more. Unless you're a seasoned cold swimmer, keep immersion under five minutes. Cold water swimming, while linked with improved mood and even fewer menopausal symptoms, still carries risks, like hormonal disruption or hypothermia, if overdone.

Think of cold exposure as a supportive reset, not a competition. A little can leave you clear-headed, energized, and resilient. Too much can tip your system the other way. Gradual progression, careful listening, and plenty of warmth afterward are the real secrets.

Infrared Sauna

Saunas have been used for thousands of years as places of warmth, cleansing, and renewal. From the Roman baths I once visited in Bath to today's modern infrared cabins, heat has long been a ritual for both physical and emotional restoration. The soothing warmth relaxes the nervous system, eases anxiety, and creates space to reconnect body, mind, and spirit.

For women in midlife, infrared saunas offer a gentler, more supportive option than traditional high-heat versions. As hormones fluctuate, recovery often slows, inflammation increases, and the nervous system becomes more sensitive. While overdoing it in a traditional sauna can sometimes stress the body, infrared heat penetrates more deeply at a lower temperature, promoting cellular detoxification without overwhelming your system.

The benefits are wide-ranging: improved circulation, reduced stiffness in muscles and joints, lighter moods, clearer skin, and even support for heart health through better blood flow and help lower blood pressure. Many women also notice relief from brain fog and hormone-related sluggishness, along with a gentle boost to metabolism.

I've personally used an infrared sauna for over twenty years and consider it one of my go-to recovery rituals. Still, I've learned to listen carefully. On days when my energy is low or fatigue is strong, I give myself permission to skip it. When I do use the sauna, I start slow, beginning with 10 minutes and working up to 30 minutes, two or three times a week. Hydration is non-negotiable, as you'll sweat deeply, and your body will thank you for replenishing lost fluids.

A word of caution: if you're experiencing frequent hot flashes or severe fatigue, start with shorter, cooler sessions, or wait until symptoms ease. Heat can sometimes intensify hot flashes or drain energy when your system is already under strain. The key is to go gently, listen to your body, and use the sauna as a supportive, restorative tool rather than another demand.

Bodywork

Massage

Massage can be a game-changer for recovery and everyday life. Safe, nurturing touch signals to your body it's okay to relax. Breathing deepens, heart rate slows, stress hormones drop, and muscles soften. Tight or overused tissues release, easing pain, improving movement, and reducing the stiffness many midlife women feel with hormonal changes and stress. It also boosts circulation and lymph flow, delivering oxygen and nutrients more effectively to support healing.

Massage pairs beautifully with other therapies, from physiotherapy to post-injury care. Techniques like lymphatic drainage reduce swelling and inflammation, while deep tissue work loosens tight fascia and muscles that might otherwise compress nerves and restrict blood flow. Even deeper layers benefit when surface tension is released.

And then there's the self-care piece. With deadlines, family demands, teenagers, aging parents, and the relentlessness of daily life, taking time for yourself often slips to the bottom of the list. Many clients tell me massage feels "too indulgent" or "too expensive." Yet we'll easily spend on shoes, takeaways, or everyone else's needs. Massage is a nourishing reminder: *you matter, too.*

The best massage is the one that meets your body where it is that day, whether that's relaxation to soothe stress, deep tissue to work through tightness, lymphatic drainage to ease swelling, or sports massage to support recovery. Each style has its place, and the right one will leave you feeling lighter, freer, and more able to move through life with ease.

Types of Massage

- Remedial/Therapeutic Massage. Targets specific injuries, pain, or movement dysfunctions rather than treating the whole body. It helps restore mobility, ease tension, and improve posture. One approach I love is Hellerwork Structural Integration, which combines myofascial release with movement education to realign the body and leave you feeling lighter, stronger, and more connected.

- Relaxation Massage. Sometimes called Swedish massage, this style uses long, flowing strokes to calm the nervous system and boost circulation. Gentle and soothing, it's the perfect choice when you're stressed, overwhelmed, or simply craving deep relaxation.

- Manual Lymphatic Drainage. A gentle, slow massage designed to stimulate the lymphatic system and clear excess fluid or toxins. It's especially helpful after illness, surgery, or during periods of inflammation or fatigue. I found it invaluable during my own recovery from burnout, when deep pressure was too much but I still needed circulation and support.

- Sports Massage. Designed to support performance and recovery, this massage focuses on tight or overused areas, like shoulders, hips, or neck. It improves mobility, eases stiffness, and can help prevent injury, whether you're training hard, sitting at a desk all day, or juggling the physical demands of daily life.

Acupuncture

Used for thousands of years to support the body's natural healing processes, acupuncture is especially helpful during menopause. Rooted in traditional Chinese medicine, acupuncture works by stimulating specific points on the body to restore the flow of energy, or Qi. From a

Western perspective, it may help regulate the nervous system, reduce inflammation, and trigger the release of feel-good endorphins. During midlife, acupuncture can be a deeply supportive tool for symptoms like fatigue, hot flashes, night sweats, mood swings, insomnia, and even anxiety. For many women, it creates a deep sense of calm and helps reestablish inner balance without relying solely on medication.

I've seen amazing results from regular acupuncture. I visit a Chinese doctor who uses acupuncture to help balance my energy and blood pressure. During some of my worst fatigue periods, weekly acupuncture sessions were what kept me from becoming completely bedridden. They kept me grounded when nothing else seemed to help and became an essential part of my recovery and upkeep routine.

Chiropractic and Osteopathy

As we move through perimenopause and menopause, stiffness, joint pain, posture shifts, and even recurring headaches can become more common. Treatments like chiropractic care and osteopathy can be invaluable for maintaining alignment, easing discomfort, and preventing structural imbalances as we age. Both aim to improve movement and function, but they work in slightly different ways.

Chiropractic care focuses on spinal alignment and nervous system regulation. It can reduce tension, improve posture, and support nervous system health, especially helpful for neck pain, back tightness, or stress-related headaches. Many women also find it helps balance energy, easing that "wired and tired" feeling.

Osteopathy takes a whole-body approach, using hands-on techniques to release restrictions in joints, muscles, fascia, and connective tissue. It can be particularly beneficial for hormone-related discomforts like bloating, pelvic tightness, digestive changes, or fluid retention. Many women find it complements other therapies beautifully, helping them feel more grounded and in tune with their bodies.

Personally, I've found that regular chiropractic care, usually once a month, acts like a reset button for my structure and energy. When I stay consistent, I notice fewer aches, better posture, and more freedom in both my workouts and everyday life.

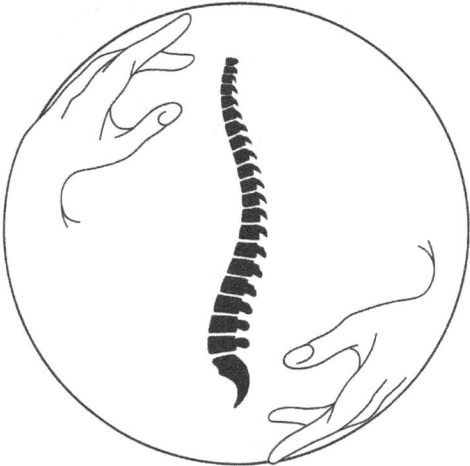

CHAPTER 15

Reset Stress and Restore Sleep

"Sleep is not an optional lifestyle luxury. Sleep is a non-negotiable biological necessity."

– MATTHEW WALKER

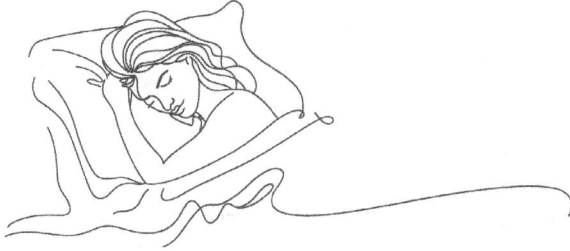

Repair with Rest

This chapter is your official permission slip to pause, exhale, and reset.

Let's start with this truth: You deserve deep rest. Not just clocking eight hours, but waking up with a sense of wholeness, the kind of rest that lets you meet life's curveballs without crumbling. The kind of sleep that softens your sharp edges and steadies your heart.

And here's the good news: Your nervous system can be rewired. Your body wants to sleep. Your calm is not lost; it's just waiting for you to come home to it.

Sleep struggles aren't personal failings. They're physiological shifts. When estrogen takes a backseat and melatonin production drops, the path to sleep becomes a winding road. Add in modern stressors and hormonal upheaval, and your nights are suddenly filled with hot flashes, racing thoughts, and the kind of overthinking that turns bedtime into a battleground.

But here's the shift: Sleep isn't a competition. It's not another thing to master or optimize. It's a relationship with your body, your rhythm, and your nervous system. It's about creating conditions that allow you to let go.

You don't need Himalayan salt lamps and lavender diffusers in every room (though, hey, they're lovely). What you need is consistency, gentleness, and a few simple practices that signal: *You're safe now.*

Let's unpack why sleep changes during menopause, how stress hijacks your internal rhythm, and what small, sustainable steps can help you reclaim your rest. No gimmicks. No guilt. Just you giving yourself what you've always given others: care, kindness, and the chance to feel whole again. Cotton pajamas optional. But highly recommended.

The Sleep-Stress Cycle

During menopause, your circadian rhythm can start acting like it's had one too many glasses of wine. This tiny timekeeper, nestled in your hypothalamus, does more than just tell you when to sleep and wake. It regulates everything from body temperature and metabolism to hormone production and how you respond to stress. When estrogen and progesterone begin to fluctuate, your body's natural rhythm can go completely off beat.

Progesterone is nature's calming balm, while estrogen supports serotonin and melatonin, the dynamic duo responsible for emotional balance and easy, restful sleep. It's like someone's fiddling with your thermostat and dimmer switch at the same time. Cue the night sweats, restless legs, and three a.m. mental grocery lists.

Understanding Your Nervous System

Your nervous system feels every bit of this disruption. With less hormonal cushioning, your sympathetic nervous system, the one that triggers fight-or-flight, can get stuck in overdrive. Meanwhile, the parasympathetic system, responsible for rest and recovery, lingers in the background, unsure how to take the lead anymore.

This imbalance is all too familiar for many women in midlife. It makes it harder to wind down, as your body is buzzing when you crave calm, and your mind runs wild at three a.m., replaying conversations or planning your retirement when you'd rather be asleep.

Here's the good news: Once you understand what's happening, you can stop fighting your body and start working with it. Gentle, science-backed shifts, like steady evening routines, calming breathwork, and moments of stillness, remind your nervous system that it is safe to slow down. Preferably before you find yourself stress-Googling kitchen renovations at two a.m.

And as we are about to explore in more detail, rest is not an indulgence. It is essential. Small steps begin to retrain your body, helping you rediscover the natural rhythm of calm and repair that has always been within you.

Why Rest Isn't Just Nice, It's Necessary

Instead of powering you forward, pushing through leaves you wired, tired, and sometimes crying over a broken coffee mug. That's because as estrogen and progesterone decline, your nervous system becomes more sensitive.

Think of your body as having two gears:

- Sympathetic (fight-or-flight): the accelerator. It spikes adrenaline and cortisol, which is great for escaping lions; less so for traffic jams, back-to-back emails, or your 10 p.m. to-do list.

- Parasympathetic (rest-and-digest): the brake. It slows your heart, calms your mind, supports digestion, repair and hormonal balance.

With less hormonal cushioning, many midlife women get stuck pressing the accelerator. Modern stressors keep the accelerator jammed, leaving you buzzing with stress hormones, sleepless at night, foggy by day, and wondering why you feel "wired but tired."

Here's the empowering shift: You can train your nervous system to switch gears. Rest isn't indulgent; it's essential maintenance. Practices like deep breathing, gentle yoga, stretching, journaling, walking in nature, or simply sitting quietly with a cup of tea and a cuddle with your fur baby all signal safety. Even 10 minutes of doing nothing tells your body: *You can soften now.*

Rest is also about rhythm. Chronic busyness creates an addictive "stress high," but the crash is brutal. I know, because I lived that way until my body collapsed. Midlife taught me the truth: Rest isn't optional. It's survival.

Ways to Rest Your Stress Mode

Simple Nervous System Resets

The good news is you don't need hours of meditation or a retreat in Bali. Little things, done with consistency, retrain your body to rest and heal. Here are a few to weave into your day:

- Breathe to reset. Try diaphragmatic breathing or the 4-7-8 breath (inhale for 4, hold for 7, exhale for 8). Just six slow breaths can signal to your body that the danger has passed.

- Move gently. Go for a slow walk in nature, barefoot if you can. Stretch for ten minutes or choose restorative Pilates over high intensity when your body feels tender.

- Create stillness. Light a candle, sip a warm tea, or simply watch the clouds roll by. Stillness doesn't have to be grand. It's the pause that restores.

- Soothing rituals.

  o A warm bath before bed or a splash of cold at the end of a shower.

  o Weighted blankets, soft humming or music that slows your heartbeat.

- A 3-minute reset during the day: one minute of movement, one of breathing, one of simply being.

- Connect with calm. Connection is medicine.

  - Hug someone you love for 20 seconds or longer.

  - Cuddle your pet.

  - Speak kindly to yourself in the mirror.

- Unplug to unwind. Turn off the noise, news, emails, endless scrolling. Gift yourself a tech-free hour, or even a "slow day."

- Engage your senses. Lavender on your pillow, soft music, a warm bath. Your senses are gateways back to peace.

- Practice the mini-pause. Close your eyes. Exhale fully. Do absolutely nothing for one whole minute. It's tiny, but powerful.

- Make space to just be. Sit in the sun. Doodle. Stare out the window. Remember: rest heals. Doing "nothing" is often doing the most.

Breathing Practices

Breath deserves its own spotlight because it's the fastest way to soothe your nervous system. Out with the stale air, in with the fresh. That's the essence of conscious breathing: A simple, accessible way to steady your energy, calm your mind, and come back to yourself.

So often, our breath runs on autopilot. Stress, hormones, and busyness can make it shallow, tight, or rushed. That's why midlife is the perfect moment to pause and notice. With just a few minutes of intentional breathing, you can reset your nervous system and release tension you may not even realize you're carrying.

And here's the beauty: You don't need special equipment or extra time. You can practice lying in bed, sitting in the car, or walking outside. A handful of deep, steady breaths can leave you feeling more grounded, more present, and more in control.

Whenever possible, breathe through your nose rather than your mouth. Nasal breathing naturally slows your breath, filters the air, and signals your body to relax. Resting your tongue gently on the roof of your mouth helps open your airway, improve posture, and supports calmer, more efficient breathing.

I once did a course in the Buteyko Method, and what struck me was how quickly small breathing shifts can change how you feel. By softening and slowing the breath, you can experience more open airways, steadier energy, and even improved sleep in just a few minutes. It's a beautiful reminder that the way we breathe isn't just background; it shapes our health, mood, and resilience every single day.

It's a small act with a big ripple: Your body exhales stress, your mind clears, and your heart feels lighter.

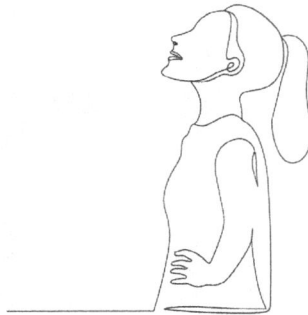

Simple Breathing Practices for Calm and Energy

- Belly Breathing (Diaphragmatic Breathing). Place one hand on your belly, one on your chest. Inhale through your nose and feel your belly rise. Exhale slowly through your mouth, making the out-breath longer than the in-breath. *Benefits: Eases stress, relaxes shoulders, and helps your body reset.*

- Pursed-Lip Breathing. Inhale through your nose, then exhale slowly through pursed lips as if blowing out a candle. *Benefits: Slows your breath, eases tension, and restores calm, especially if you feel anxious or short of breath.*

- 4-7-8 Breathing. Inhale for 4, hold for 7, exhale for 8. Repeat up to four rounds. *Benefits: Supports sleep, soothes the nervous system, and quiets a busy mind.*

- Mindful Breathing. Simply notice your breath. Feel the rise and fall of your chest, the coolness as you inhale, the warmth as you exhale. *Benefits: Anchors you in the present and softens racing thoughts.*

- Alternate Nostril Breathing (Nadi Shodhana). Close your right nostril and inhale through the left. Switch and exhale through the right. Inhale right, exhale left. Continue. *Benefits: Balances energy, sharpens focus, and calms agitation.*

A Gentle Reminder

Even two minutes of conscious breathing can shift how you feel. Try it while waiting for the kettle to boil, sitting in traffic, or before bed. Over time, your body remembers how to breathe deeply again, a quiet gift for steadier hormones, calmer days, and more peaceful nights.

Practice Makes Progress

Breathing takes practice, and the best time to start is when you're calm. When shifting hormones can trigger hot flashes, racing thoughts, and restless nights, just 5 to 10 minutes a day of intentional breathing can make a real difference. These simple practices help cool the body, calm the nervous system, and ease anxiety while also supporting better sleep and steadier energy.

Over time, your body relearns how to breathe more efficiently, a gift for hormone balance, focus, and resilience during this stage of life. Even something as small as shifting from mouth to nasal breathing can help you feel more grounded, centered, and in control. Sometimes, healing really does begin with just one mindful inhale.

As mentioned earlier in the book, both melatonin and magnesium are key players in midlife sleep balance. Melatonin is the hormone that gently whispers, "time to sleep." It naturally declines with age, which makes it harder to fall asleep and stay asleep. Since it's also a powerful antioxidant, this drop affects not only your rest but your body's recovery too. Clearly, menopause likes to multitask.

Breaking the Sleep Stress, Weight Loop

And then there's the sneaky sleep-stress-weight loop, a vicious cycle where poor sleep throws your hunger hormones off balance, ramps up cortisol (your stress-storage hormone), and leaves you craving carbs while feeling more frazzled than ever. This isn't about willpower; it's biology in a bit of a meltdown. That's why treating sleep as sacred is so essential during this stage.

Create a nighttime routine that tells your body, "It's safe to let go now." Cool your bedroom to around 65°F (18°C). Make it dark, quiet, and screen-free. Declare the hour before bed a no-news, no-email, no-texts zone. Think of it as sleep hygiene with a rebellious twist: "No, I will not reply to that Slack message. I choose sanity."

What you do during the day matters, too. Move your body early (not with a HIIT class at nine p.m.), limit caffeine to the morning, and manage stress with practices that ground you. Try going to bed at the same time every night. Your body thrives on rhythm, especially when your hormones don't.

And if you do wake up at 2 a.m. because, let's face it, you probably will sometimes, have a gentle plan ready. Light stretching, meditation, chamomile tea, or reading a dull book under soft, low light can help coax your brain back into rest mode. Remember, whatever you do, don't check your phone. That screen will reignite the mental circus faster than you can say, "Why is my ex posting cryptic memes again?"

Gentle Compassion

Understanding how your nervous system, hormones, and sleep all interact helps you move through these changes with more compassion and a little humor, too. This isn't about trying to claw your way back to the sleep you had in your thirties. It's about honoring your evolving body and creating the conditions it needs now.

Above all, be gentle with yourself. Some nights will feel blissful. Others might feel like you're starring in a reality show called *Who Needs Sleep Anyway?* But every small, intentional act, every magnesium-rich snack, every breathwork session, every screen-free wind-down, is a vote for your wellbeing. Because in midlife, rest isn't a luxury. It's your birthright. And you, my friend, are worth every ounce of care it takes to reclaim it.

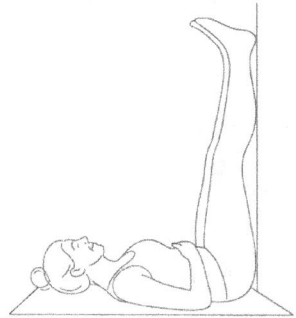

Creating Your Restorative Evening Ritual

Creating a restorative evening ritual is like building a soft runway, one that gently guides you from the chaos of the day into the deep, healing rest your body craves.

During menopause, this wind-down becomes even more crucial. Let's face it, our nervous systems now respond to disruption the way toddlers respond to skipped naps: not well.

When I first started struggling with sleep during early perimenopause, I realized my evening routine needed to start much earlier than I'd ever imagined, basically right after sunset. Our bodies are designed to begin producing melatonin as the light fades, but modern life, working late, eating late, drinking alcohol, with its blazing screens, endless streaming, and late-night scroll-athons bulldoze that signal.

That's when I discovered something I call "sunset signaling," the conscious act of dimming the lights, lighting candles, lowering the volume, and winding down with the day instead of fighting it like a caffeinated hamster.

The first secret to building your own ritual? Find your "power-down hour," that magic window two to three hours before bed when you stop pretending you're a high-functioning adult and start preparing your mind and body for rest.

It doesn't require meditating on a mountaintop. It's about simple, consistent shifts: turning off overhead lights, switching your phone to *Do Not Disturb*, putting away the to-do list, and maybe wandering around the house like a peaceful old cat.

Temperature regulation is another unsung hero. Night sweats and hot flashes are your body's protest march and ignoring them doesn't help.

One of my favorite tricks? A warm bath or shower about 90 minutes before bed. It sounds counterintuitive, but it actually triggers your body's cooling mechanisms, making it easier to fall asleep. Bonus: Add Epsom salts for a luxurious magnesium boost, calming your nervous system without another pill.

Soft rituals like these weave beautifully into your transition to sleep. A mug of chamomile or lemon balm tea. A few minutes of breathwork. Gentle stretches. These aren't indulgences; they're how you whisper to your body, "You're safe. You can let go now."

Stretching doesn't need to be fancy. Think more yawning cat than Instagram contortionist. Try child's pose, legs up the wall, or a gentle spinal twist, movements that ease you toward rest without overheating or waking your inner perfectionist.

Nutrition still plays a supporting role. Try to finish dinner at least three hours before bed so your body isn't busy digesting when it should be restoring. If you're hungry later, choose a small, calm snack, like a handful of almonds or a splash of tart cherry juice, which naturally boosts melatonin (and yes, it also feels elegantly grown-up).

Your bedroom should feel like a sanctuary, not a second office. Banish electronics (or at least hide them in a drawer), dim the lights, use blackout curtains, and aim for a cool, dark, quiet space. Essential oils, like lavender or frankincense, can be surprisingly powerful, like aromatherapy bribery for your brain.

One tiny but mighty upgrade? What you wear to bed matters. Choose breathable fabrics like cotton, bamboo, or linen. They help regulate body temperature and wick away moisture, lifesavers when hot flashes strike. Your sheets matter too. Natural fibers allow your skin to breathe so you're not peeling off a sweaty synthetic nightie like an exhausted escape artist at three a.m.

Managing stress before bed is the cherry on top. Try the 4-7-8 breathing technique (inhale for 4, hold for 7, exhale for 8). It helps shut off your brain's late-night panic radio.

And if you're prone to lying awake mentally redecorating your home or rewriting that awkward conversation from earlier? Journaling is a game-changer. A quick brain dump, or jotting down three good things from your day, can clear the clutter and help you settle.

Remember, sleep isn't just a break, it's your body's prime time for healing. It's when your hormones rebalance, your mind processes memories, and your body stitches itself back together. The key is consistency over perfection. Start with one or two rituals that feel good and build from there. What works one month might need tweaking the next, and that's okay.

Think of your evening routine as a menu, not a checklist. You're the chef. Your circadian rhythm loves routine, like a toddler loves a bedtime story, and a regular sleep schedule trains your body to rest more easily. I aim for lights out by 10.30 p.m. and wake around seven a.m. That eight to nine hours aren't a luxury. It's essential. Especially during menopause, your body is working overtime to restore balance. Deep, consistent sleep supports hormone regulation, brain function, mood, and energy for the day ahead.

We often think of sleep as one long snooze, but it runs in cycles. The first half of the night is all about physical repair, healing tissues, building muscle, supporting your immune system. The second half is where the emotional magic happens, processing memories, tidying up mental clutter, and realizing you don't actually need to rejoin that WhatsApp group.

Most midlife women thrive on seven to nine hours of sleep per night. Less than six hours regularly? That can spike cortisol, wreck your blood sugar balance, and make life feel like a nonstop soap opera (spoiler: it's exhausting).

That's why prioritizing a nourishing nighttime ritual isn't just about getting sleep. It's about giving your body, mind, and spirit the nightly reset they need to thrive.

Some nights will be smooth.

Others will be chaos.

Progress, not perfection.

Pajamas on. Phone off.

Self-compassion fully activated

You've got this!

Sleep Tip: Don't Force It

Still awake after 20 minutes? Get up. Make a cozy nest on the couch with a blanket and a gentle book (no screens, no Netflix binges). When sleepiness creeps back, return to bed. It's like house-training your brain: Bed is for snoozing, not three a.m. grocery lists.

If you're suffering from hot flashes, get up and take a cool shower or use a damp cloth to lower your body temperature, then change into light, breathable nightwear such as cotton.

You don't need to do every step every night. Think of this as a gentle menu, not a to-do list. The magic is in creating rituals that feel grounding and repeatable, helping your body associate these cues with rest. Over time, you'll find yourself not just falling asleep more easily but actually looking forward to this precious time to unwind and reconnect with yourself.

Nap Like a Pro: The Power of the 20-Minute Reset

Feeling like your brain has gone offline around 3 p.m.? You're not alone, and you're not lazy. That mid-afternoon energy dip is biological, not a personal failing. In fact, our bodies naturally follow a circadian rhythm that includes a dip in alertness between one and three p.m. (no, it's not just the aftermath of lunch or your morning coffee wearing off).

So, instead of powering through in a fog, consider this: what if the best productivity hack isn't another espresso or pushing through, but a nap?

Yep, I'm talking about the grown-up version of nap time. A 15- to 20-minute nap can do wonders. It boosts alertness, improves memory and focus, and can even reduce cortisol levels (hello, calmer nervous system). And here's the kicker: Elite athletes do it. I recently watched a documentary where top-tier athletes were prescribed short naps after lunch as part of their recovery protocols. Why? Because those little power naps help muscle repair, improve reaction times, and support overall performance, physically and mentally.

The key here is to nap smart. Keep it short, around 20 minutes or less. Any longer, and you risk sliding into deeper sleep stages, which can leave you waking up groggy (a.k.a. the dreaded nap hangover).

Aim to rest between one p.m. and three p.m. This aligns with your natural dip in energy and won't interfere with nighttime sleep. Create a calm space. Dim the lights, pop on an eye mask, and get cozy. Even just lying down and closing your eyes for 10 to 20 minutes can calm your nervous system.

If you're in midlife and navigating fluctuating hormones, hot flashes, disrupted sleep, or adrenal fatigue, a short nap can be like a mini reset button. It's not indulgent; it's intelligent recovery. You're not being lazy. You're restoring your brain, body, and mood.

Think of it as a 20-minute gift to yourself. A reset for your mind, a boost for your body, and a gentle reminder that sometimes doing less is the smartest thing you can do.

Signs You Need a Rest Day

Rest days aren't a weakness. They're part of your progress. In midlife, your body often needs more recovery than before, especially as hormones shift and stress stacks up. If you're feeling "off," it's not always about pushing harder. Sometimes, the bravest move is to pause.

Here are a few clear signals your body might be asking for a break:

1. Persistent soreness. A little post-workout ache is normal, but if it lingers for days, your muscles haven't fully repaired. That's your cue to rest.

2. Deep fatigue. Being tired is one thing; feeling drained before you even start moving is another. If simple tasks feel heavy, it's time to reset.

3. Aches and pains. Ongoing joint or muscle pain can mean overuse or inflammation. Listen now so you don't end up sidelined later.

4. Mood dips. Burnout doesn't just show up in your body; it shows up in your mood. Irritability, anxiety, or feeling flat can all be your nervous system waving a white flag.

5. Poor sleep. Overexercising can backfire, raising cortisol and leaving you wired at night instead of deeply rested.

6. Sluggish performance. When workouts feel harder than usual or progress stalls, the problem isn't effort; it's recovery.

7. Weakened immunity. If you're picking up every bug going around, it might be a sign your body needs downtime to repair and strengthen defenses.

8. Low motivation. When exercise or even daily activities feel more like punishment than joy, rest can rekindle your spark.

One of the tools I love is creating a personal energy map to help you tune in. Notice when you naturally feel alive and switched on and when you tend to crash. Pay attention to how different movements or even everyday events shift your mood and sleep.

Your energy won't look the same every day, and it will definitely change across your menopause journey. That's normal. The trick is to stay flexible and keep adjusting. When you start lining up your daily activities with your body's signals, you discover a deeper strength and a more sustainable vibrancy.

Think of it as partnering with your body instead of pushing against it.

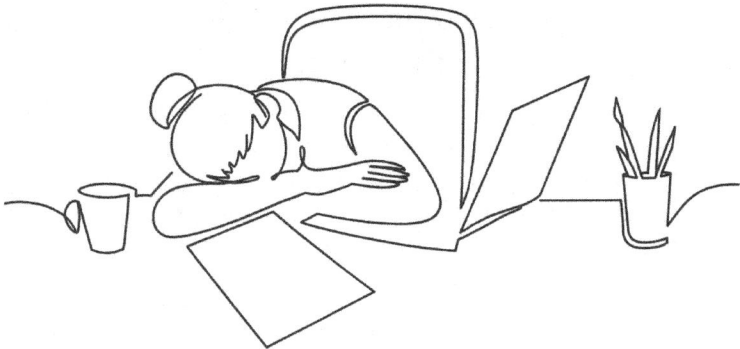

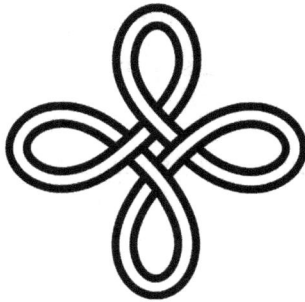

Pillar Five –
Connection, Joy, and Purpose

"Make connections, make friends, join communities, and really honor yourself. You're getting ready to make that transition to menopause, so pay attention to where you're at emotionally, physically, and mentally. I believe that it's a privilege to get older. Not everyone gets older."

– CAMERON DIAZ, ACTRESS

When midlife has flipped the script and leaves you more as a wilting wallflower than an abundantly thriving rose, it may seem impossible to move beyond merely surviving toward a life of joyful abandon and motivation, no matter how much rest, recovery, healthy food, and nourishing movement you give your body. Chances are, you'll need a little extra boost to start thriving again.

CHAPTER 16

Relationships Support and Connections

"Here's what I know: I'm a better person at fifty than I was at forty-eight... and better at fifty-two than I was at fifty. I'm calmer, easier to live with. All this stuff is in my soul forever. Just don't get lazy. Work at your relationships all the time. Take care of friendships, hold people you love close to you, take advantage of birthdays to celebrate fiercely. It's the worrying–not the years themselves–that will make you less of a woman."

– PATTI LABELLE

This quote feels like a deep exhale. It reminds us that midlife is not a loss but a deepening. Patti LaBelle captures something many of us quietly hope is true: that with time comes wisdom, grace, and a greater understanding of what truly matters. It's not the years that wear us down; it's the pressure, worry, and neglect of our own joy.

Her words are a perfect way to start this chapter because if there's one thing worth reclaiming fiercely and tenderly, it's our sense of intimacy, both with our partners and ourselves.

Let's begin with the conversation that often gets overlooked in menopause talks: sex, sensuality, and connection.

This phase of life brings significant physical, emotional, and relational changes. Many women feel detached from their bodies or partners and are uncertain about how to handle changes in desire or body confidence.

This chapter is an invitation to courageously come home to yourself again with compassion and some curiosity. Because you still deserve pleasure, connection, and that fierce kind of love.

Self-Love

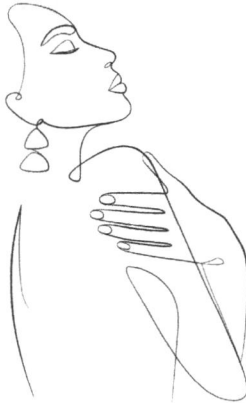

I look back at photos of myself in my twenties, thirties, and forties and see a body that was lean, firm, and toned. And yet, I remember thinking at the time that I was "fat." We are often so hard on ourselves, quick to spot flaws instead of celebrating our uniqueness.

As we weave our way into our fifties, sixties, and beyond, our bodies may not look the way they once did. But every wrinkle, gray hair, scars, so-called imperfections are actually signs of resilience, strength, and a life well lived. Without them, we wouldn't be who we are today. This season invites us to flip the script, to notice not just our faults but our powers. Our superpowers. The knowledge and wisdom we now hold can't be measured in a mirror. They are gifts we can share in ways we couldn't before.

Before we talk about relationships with friends, partners, family, or colleagues, we need to pause and talk about the one relationship that underpins them all: the one you have with yourself.

Self-love isn't about quick fixes or Instagram clichés (though a long soak in a bubble bath can be a beautiful way to unwind); it's about learning to meet your own needs with the same generosity you've spent years pouring into everyone else. Too often, midlife women find themselves running on empty, giving endlessly but rarely stopping to refill their own well.

Your body has been working for you your whole life. It has carried you through every season, every challenge, and every joy. Be grateful for it. It doesn't define your worth or your intelligence. It's a reflection of how well you care for yourself.

So today, ask yourself, "What would make me feel loved and supported right now?" Maybe it's saying no without guilt, cooking yourself a nourishing meal, walking barefoot in the grass, buying yourself a beautiful bunch of flowers, booking a relaxing massage, or phoning a friend who always makes you laugh. Small acts of care send a powerful signal to your nervous system: *I matter, too.*

Sometimes, self-love looks less like a treat and more like a boundary. Saying no to what drains you creates space to say yes to what truly lights you up. Even tiny daily anchors: a quiet tea before the household wakes, three deep breaths before opening your laptop, or a walk at sunset with your fur baby, can remind you that your wellbeing counts.

Another gentle practice: Instead of scanning the mirror for flaws, try looking at yourself the way you'd look at someone you love. A soft smile, a kind thought, even a whispered "thank you" to your body for carrying you this far. Look deep into your own eyes and see the beautiful, unique soul looking back at you. It might feel awkward at first, but over time, it shifts the way you see yourself, from critic to being your own cheerleader.

And if you forget some days? That's okay, too; don't beat yourself up. We're human, not machines. We can be our own worst critics. Self-love grows when you extend yourself the same kindness and compassion you would give a dear friend. And when you love yourself enough to honor your needs, every other relationship in your life begins to shift in the best possible way.

The Power of Sisterhood

Have you ever noticed how, when a group of women gather, the noise level skyrockets? The energy lifts, and the urge to share, talk, laugh, and connect takes over. It's healing at any time of day, and in midlife, it's vital. We need to find ways to connect and share. It boosts joy and stimulates our happy hormones.

One of the greatest gifts of my life is the bond I share with my girlfriends. We've known each other since we were five years old. So, by the time we turned fifty, we had celebrated forty-five incredible years of friendship. These women are more than friends; they are my chosen family. We called ourselves "The Fabulous Fifties" when we reached that milestone and began taking holidays together to mark each new decade. The moment we pile into a car or hop on a plane, it's like time stands still. We pick up right where we left off, belly-laughing until we cry, sharing everything from skincare tips to life's deepest challenges and biggest triumphs. We don't see each other every day, but they are my soul sisters.

Having this kind of connection during menopause has been a lifeline for me. These friendships help you feel seen, supported, and maybe, just maybe, keep you a little more sane in the chaos. In a time of life when everything feels like it's shifting, they help me feel grounded. Now, as we approach our sixties, we're wondering whether we will become "The Sensational Sixties" or perhaps 'The Fabulous Swifties' (much to our children's embarrassment, as they roll their eyes every time our WhatsApp group, 'Fabulous 50s,' lights up their screens). No matter what we call ourselves, one thing is clear: This sisterhood is pure gold. It gives me a deep sense of belonging and reminds me that I'm not alone on this wild, beautiful ride through midlife.

So, if you don't have a ride-or-die crew yet, create one! Join a club, start ladies-only dinners, form a book club, start a walking group, or join a tennis team. It doesn't matter what you're doing as long as you're connecting, sharing, and laughing. That energy and those endorphins? They're exactly the kind of joy your midlife hormones crave.

Pleasure on Your Terms

As estrogen and testosterone levels decline, symptoms like vaginal dryness, reduced libido, or discomfort during sex may occur. These changes are happening, but they don't have to define your experience. With support, hormone therapy, vaginal estrogen, lubricants, and honest communication, many of these issues can be managed or even reversed. Your body still deserves pleasure. You still deserve to feel sensual and vibrantly alive.

Sexual well-being is more than just biology. For many, the biggest shift is internal: reclaiming personal desire, redefining intimacy, and letting go of outdated beliefs about what sex "should" look like. Maybe intimacy now means sharing stories or rediscovering the joy of solo pleasure. This is your moment to ask, "What do I want? What feels good right now, in this body, in this chapter of my life?"

Midlife often changes how we see our bodies. Yes, there may be softness and wrinkles, but there's also wisdom and liberation. The more you focus on how your body feels rather than how it looks, the more you reclaim your sensuality on your terms. You are allowed to crave pleasure. To seek it out. To define it. This isn't the end of your sexuality. It's an invitation to rewrite it with honesty, curiosity, and joy. Be gentle. Be truthful with yourself and with those who love you. Your pleasure matters. Your body is still yours. This is not the ending. It's an unfolding.

This next chapter is yours to shape, and how you experience pleasure, intimacy, or connection is entirely up to you. For some women, it's a relief to leave behind the pressures of fertility and redefine this season on their own terms. That might mean embracing new forms of intimacy, focusing their creative energy elsewhere, or simply choosing to pause or even let go of sex altogether. The beauty is you get to choose.

Intimacy doesn't have to mean sex; it can be found in deep conversations, shared laughter, quiet companionship, touch without expectation, acts of care, mutual respect, emotional vulnerability, or simply being fully present with one another. Conversations can be one of the most powerful ways to stay connected, whether you're reminiscing about shared memories, exploring dreams for the future, or simply talking honestly about how you feel. Many women say that redefining intimacy in midlife brought them closer to their partners. It's about connection, not performance.

Sharing with Your Partner

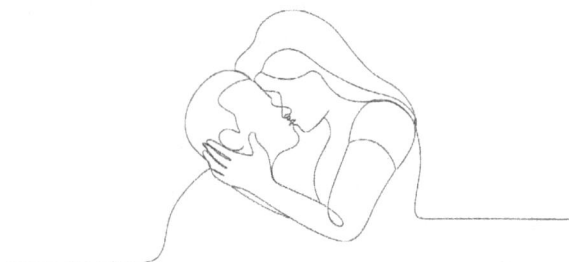

Menopause doesn't happen in isolation. It ripples out into your relationships, with your partner, children, friends, and aging parents. But many women go through this transition quietly, feeling like they have to hold it all together. You don't have to do it alone. Start by opening up to the people closest to you, especially your partner.

For many partners, this time is confusing. They can't understand what you're experiencing if you don't share it with them. They're not mind readers. They may look at you and quietly wonder, "Who is this stranger in my house?" Suddenly, the person they love seems distant, turning down intimacy, or snapping over small things. Without context, they feel confused or even rejected. The once calm, affectionate version of you may withdraw or easily upset. You both need new ways of staying connected.

Honest, open-hearted conversations about your symptoms and emotional shifts are essential to help your partner understand. Imagine how bewildering it must be when the person they love suddenly pulls away, not because they don't care, but because they're drenched in a puddle of night sweats, feeling exhausted, overstimulated, and overwhelmed. The last thing on your mind in that moment is cuddling, let alone sex. And when intimacy does come up, vaginal dryness or pain can make the experience feel more distressing than pleasurable.

In fact, research shows that a significant number of breakups and divorces happen during the menopausal transition, often because emotional and physical changes go unspoken. Relationships can quietly unravel just when support is most needed.

Try beginning with something simple and vulnerable, like: "I'm going through hormonal changes that are affecting my energy, my body, and how I feel. I still care deeply about us, but I may need different things right now." Let them know how they can support you, whether that means giving you space, holding your hand, listening without trying to fix things, or simply being present through it all.

If intimacy has become painful, it's okay to say: "I'm finding sex uncomfortable at the moment. Can we try using a vaginal lubricant or estrogen cream? Or maybe we can connect in other ways, like holding hands on a beach walk, or just lying close together. I want to feel close to you, even if it looks a little different for now."

You can also explore new rituals together. "What if we had a weekly date night again? Got out of the house, talked about something other than stress, and remembered how we used to connect before kids, mortgages, and work took over?"

This season invites a deeper kind of intimacy. It may not look the same as it did in your thirties, and that's okay. What matters is you keep choosing each other, creating a safe, evolving space where both of you can grow, connect, and feel seen.

If you find it hard to explain everything, invite them to read a chapter of this book, especially the one on hormones and intimacy. It could be the bridge that helps them understand your experience and meet you with empathy.

Menopause may last several years. That's a long time to pretend or push problems under the rug. But with open-hearted communication and a shared commitment to connection, this can become one of the most honest and meaningful chapters in your relationship.

With Our Children

If we don't talk to our daughters or sons about menopause, how will they ever understand it when it's their turn or support someone going through it?

Growing up, my mother never mentioned menopause. Neither did my older sisters. When it hit me, I was blindsided. I didn't know what was happening or whether what I was experiencing was normal. That silence made me feel isolated and unprepared. And I know I'm not alone in that.

We can break that cycle.

Talking to your children about menopause doesn't have to be a formal sit-down conversation. In fact, the most powerful moments often happen casually when you're in the car, at the dinner table, on a walk, or when you're fanning yourself mid-hot flash.

You might simply say: "My hormones are changing, and it means I get tired, teary, or overwhelmed sometimes. But it's a normal part of life, and I'm learning how to look after myself." That one sentence plants a seed. For your daughter, especially, it models something she may never have seen: A woman honoring her body's transitions instead of hiding them, pushing through, or pretending she's fine. You're showing her what self-awareness and self-care actually look like. That's a legacy worth passing on.

With younger children, keep it simple and observational: "Sometimes, I get really hot, or I need more rest. My body is changing, just like everyone's does in different seasons of life."

With teens, especially those going through puberty, you can connect the dots: "What you're going through now is puberty: your body adjusting to hormones and changing into adulthood. What I'm going through is kind of the reverse: my body is adjusting again, just in a different way."

The goal isn't to give them a biology lesson. It's to normalize the conversation. Share what you're doing to support yourself, whether it's magnesium tea at night, your walk after dinner, or why you don't schedule much in the evenings anymore. These small moments help them understand that menopause is natural, and that tuning in and caring for your body is something to be proud of, not hidden.

If they ask questions, that's a good thing. And if they catch you off guard, it's completely fine to say, "That's a great question. I want to think about how to explain it well." Keep the door open for an ongoing conversation, not a one-time lecture.

Talking about menopause is not just for you, it's for them. You're giving your children a different narrative, one based in honesty, curiosity, and compassion. And one day, when they, or someone they love, face the same transition, they'll remember your openness. They'll feel more informed, more supported, and far less alone.

With Colleagues and Bosses

Menopause doesn't just influence our private lives; it also impacts our workplace. Brain fog during a meeting, fatigue after a sleepless night, or sudden hot flashes in the middle of a presentation can feel exposing and even embarrassing. Too often, women suffer in silence, fearing judgment for being a woman or aging, when what's really needed is understanding and support.

Research shows that around ten percent of women actually leave the workforce due to severe menopausal symptoms. That's a lot of women stepping away at the peak of their careers simply because workplaces haven't adapted.

Having honest conversations doesn't mean oversharing. It means asking for the small adjustments that help you show up true to yourself, without the extra load of pretending everything is fine. It might begin by talking with a trusted colleague: "I've been experiencing some changes that affect my energy and focus at times. I'm working on ways to manage them, but I'd appreciate some flexibility when I need it."

Practical adjustments, like flexible scheduling, a desk fan, air conditioning, or a quick break, can make a world of difference. I know this firsthand. At the peak of my hot flashes, I once had to pause mid-Pilates session, drenched in sweat and unable to think straight. A quick cold shower helped, but installing air conditioning in my studio was the real game changer, for me and for my clients, many of whom were navigating the same stage of life.

For managers and team leaders, kindness, respect, and a listening ear can transform workplace culture. Normalizing menopause at work doesn't just help one woman; it sets the tone for the whole workplace. It tells every employee that humanity matters as much as productivity.

If you worry about stigma, remember this: Change often begins with one brave voice. By advocating for yourself, you may open the door for others who are struggling quietly. Menopause isn't the end of your professional story. It can be the start of showing up with more authenticity, strength, and resilience than ever before. And when colleagues and bosses meet you with empathy, you're reminded you don't have to carry this alone, at home or at work.

Support in the workplace isn't about special treatment; it's about fairness, inclusion, and recognizing that midlife women bring enormous value when they're supported in the ways they need.

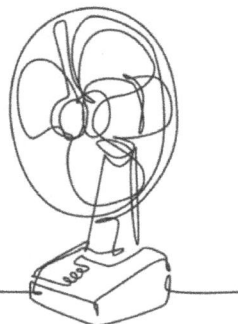

CHAPTER 17

Reclaim Your Energy and Joy

"You must be willing to let go of the life you have planned so as to have the life that is waiting for us"

– ECKHART TOLLE.

I had this revelation on the same day as my sitting-down, teaching-Pilates moment that turned everything around. Later that afternoon, walking my four-legged wellness coach, Stan, I reached a familiar set of stairs. Usually, I'd fly up them two at a time, feeling like an off-duty Nike ambassador. But that day, they felt like Mount Everest. Halfway up, breathless and heavy-legged, I paused. And for once, instead of pushing through, I listened. That night, I picked up my journal and mapped my energy patterns.

It looked like a freeway at rush hour: stop-start all the way. The biggest crash surprised me. It always came after my intense swim sessions. When I asked my coach for advice, he served up the classic gem, "Just toss some more rolled oats in your smoothie." Got to love the one-size-fits-all carb fix. But that scribble session was my turning point. I was pushing my body too hard in every area of my life, with long training sessions that were too frequent and too intense, without rest. I was burning the candle at both ends, juggling a demanding professional life with twelve-hour days and an always-on social calendar, just as I had always done. I was stuck in the habit of doing more, multitasking, and trying to squeeze as much as possible into every day. Sound familiar? What I really needed was more life balance, tuning into my well-being, and giving myself permission to take time for me, and adding restorative movement, nourishing meals, and real rest.

As my eyes opened, I saw a new phase in my life beginning. I stopped fighting my body and started working with it. I swapped punishing hour-long cardio for 20-minute strength bursts, added restorative Pilates and slow walks in nature, and (this was the hardest part) allowed myself time to rest without guilt.

Protecting my energy also meant setting my own boundaries and not overcommitting. I slowly learned to say "no" to the things that drained me, like social plans, work obligations, or the constant pressure to always show up for everyone else so that I had the space to truly recover. It wasn't easy at first, as I was so used to stretching myself thin and living on the adrenaline high of trying to have it all. But over time, I realized these weren't walls to shut people out; they were gentle fences that protected my energy, my rest, and my well-being. When I started to honor my limits and voice my needs, it gave others the chance to step in and support me. And that was a powerful reminder that my health and happiness matter just as much as anyone else's.

I started coaching differently by taking longer breaks during the day to re-energize and show up fully for my clients. Instead of working harder, I tuned in. Instead of scheduling workouts during energy dips, I learned to align with my natural highs. I replaced hustle with harmony.

Menopause is a signal to evolve. Your energy now deserves your respect. Your movement should nourish your spirit, and your motivation should no longer respond to barking trainers or exhausting sessions. It's about focusing on what fills your cup. Add some sunshine and, my personal favorite, blast your feel-good playlist while moving however your body wants to. It's about joy.

Take a spontaneous walk on the beach. Surprise someone you love with a gift of flowers. This is about reclaiming curiosity and connection to yourself, finding delight along the way. Your task is to rediscover the authentic, radiant you. Because reclaiming your mojo begins when you honor who you are today, with all the softness, strength, wisdom, and sass you've earned.

And if your spark is buried under laundry and life admin, it's time to start digging. As well-known author Florence King beautifully said, "A woman must wait for her ovaries to die before she can get her rightful personality back." Honestly? She has a point. There's something wonderfully freeing about stepping into postmenopause without the monthly rollercoaster. It's like coming home to yourself clear-headed and finally entirely on your own terms. And, darling, you're just getting started.

The Creative Spark

Here's the thing about menopause: Yes, it can bring night sweats, moods that swing harder than a roller coaster on loop, and sleep so patchy it makes you question every life choice, but it also brings something wildly underrated: space.

Space to breathe. Space to reflect. Space to be yourself. And surprise, space to rediscover that creative spark you might have buried somewhere between school drop-offs, board meetings, and an overflowing laundry basket. For many women, this desire for creativity seems to appear out of nowhere. And not in a "maybe I'll knit a scarf" way, but a deep, soulful urge to create something—anything—that isn't a meal or a to-do list. It's like your inner artist has been napping under a pile of permission slips and PTA notices, and now she's stretching, yawning, and asking, "So, what now?"

Research shows creative expression lowers cortisol, boosts mood, and even improves immune function. This is all proof that making art at midlife, however messy, is medicine.

For me, it started with a 3 a.m. wake-up, bless you, night sweats. I wandered into the garage, opened a crusty tube of paint, and somewhere between the color, the mess, and the freedom, I felt myself return.

Art has always been part of my language. My mom taught me to paint when I was little, and it quickly became my most natural form of expression. As someone with dyslexia, reading and writing were often frustrating growing up. But give me a paintbrush or a camera, and something clicks, literally. Art gives me a voice when words are hard to find.

I went on to study fine arts, earning a Bachelor of Fine Arts and a Master's in Photography. Even now, when I reconnect with that creative part of my brain, it feels like plugging back into my femininity. It softens the sharp edges of my life. It unravels the tightness that comes from constant doing. And I've seen that same magic spark in other women, too.

Take Amanda a high-powered corporate client, who was completely exhausted. She was drained and felt disconnected. She swore she wasn't creative, but one day, she suddenly mentioned a fascination with photography. We started her creative practice small, just by noticing light and shadow during her lunchtime walks. A few months later, she was taking beautiful portraits of her grandkids and glowing as if she'd reconnected with a long-lost part of herself. And here's the beautiful truth: There are no rules. You don't have to be Frida Kahlo. All you need is curiosity and maybe a willingness to get a little messy.

Grief. Rage. Joy. Longing. Confusion. That strange mix of wonder and WTAF that perimenopause throws at us daily? It all fits. Pour it out into something. Laugh about it. Move it through you by dancing, writing, or painting. This is the midlife remix: a time to listen. Don't let the fear of what other people might say stop you. Yes, someone might raise an eyebrow and whisper, "She's lost her marbles." Let them! You aren't doing it for them; you're doing it because it lights you up. Joy is reason enough. As Lady Gaga says, "Don't ever let a soul in the world tell you that you can't be exactly who you are." Because maybe, just maybe, this chapter of life isn't about slowing down. It's about showing up differently, more boldly, more honestly, and with a whole lot more glitter glue or compost, if that's more your jam.

So, go ahead, pick up the camera, the pen, the fabric, or the brush. Or turn on your favorite playlist and sing into a hairbrush. Because menopause might just be the most creative, rebellious, and permission-filled chapter of your life. And if your old inner monologue has been looping, "I'm too tired, old, or busy, and not creative enough," it's time for a rewrite. Those old stories may have kept you safe, but also small. Now they're just walls, and your mojo can't breathe behind walls. What if you tried this instead? "It's not too late. I've lived enough to finally begin, on my terms."

> *"Whether you think you can, or you think you can't, you're right."*
>
> **– HENRY FORD.**

This one always reminds me of my dad. He had a saying I'll never forget: "There's no such thing as can't." At the time, I didn't realize how much that mindset would shape me. But now I see it clearly: What you believe is everything. Once I stopped telling myself I was broken, too tired, or too far gone, and started believing I could rebuild my energy, find balance, and feel strong again, everything began to shift. Not overnight, but steadily. Change can feel scary. It's like walking an unknown path, but that's where growth begins. I gave myself permission to try new things, to change my story, and to do life a different way, on my terms. And that changed everything. What if you let yourself believe you could, too?

What Lights You Up

Midlife cracked me open with grief, enormous change, and the kind of transitions that shook the ground beneath me. Out of those lessons came a deeper honoring of every part of who I am: the coach who encourages women to move and nourish their bodies, the Pilates instructor and personal trainer who helps others feel strong and connected, the photographer who plays with light, color, and emotion to capture stories, and the gardener who finds peace in the soil, planting with intention and harvesting food with my own hands. Watching seeds sprout and flourish into both beauty and nourishment feels like a mirror of my own life: fragile at times, yet deeply resilient. Whether I create through movement, imagery, food, or nature, I return to my body, my breath, and the simple gift of presence.

For me, it is not only about what I do. It is about truth and what brings me joy. I love what I do for a living, and I honestly cannot imagine doing anything I do not love. That sense of purpose keeps me steady and energized, even during the toughest times.

Opening my new venues and launching *Your Menopause Balance* were significant leaps of faith. Both expanded my creativity and pushed the limits of what I believed I could do. They challenged long-held beliefs about myself, especially those formed as a girl with dyslexia, told by a school career advisor that I was not smart enough to take my exams and should just leave school.

Well... I wrote this book.

And every page is proof that we're never too far behind, never too late to begin again. This book is a quiet revolution, a reclaiming of voice, vision, and possibility.

Your Space, Your Story

Creativity isn't just about what you create; it's about how you live. It's how you curate your space, wardrobe, and rituals. I've transformed my home into a cozy, French-country-inspired sanctuary, filled with collected art, tactile textures, and colors that make my heart sing.

I share my mom's passion for art and culture, and we often visit local galleries together, especially when there's an international exhibition featuring inspiring artists like Vincent van Gogh, Paul Cézanne, or Pablo Picasso. My mom always says that going to a brilliantly curated art exhibition is "like sipping on a glass of expensive champagne." I couldn't agree more. I find joy not only in creating art but also in collecting it.

Surrounding myself with pieces that inspire me helps create a space I truly love, a space that reflects who I am, sparks creativity, and feels deeply personal. Whether it's a bold painting, a delicate sketch, or a quirky sculpture, these touches breathe life into any room. Your space should feel like a haven, a place to truly rest and relax, not a storage unit of the past. Let it reflect you now, the woman you're becoming, not just the one you've been.

Even if you share your space, you can still add corners of soulfulness. Maybe it's a single candle on your desk, a favorite photo, or a throw that makes you smile. Tiny creative rebellions count.

My friend Odette lives in a spotless, minimalist home, but one room is hers alone. Her own sanctuary with a cozy armchair and soft throws, candles and incense, shelves of favorite books, an heirloom piece, and her yoga mat and roller ready to go. It's where she stretches, journals, sips tea, or simply sits in stillness. Yours doesn't have to be a whole room; a deck chair or snug window nook will do. Anywhere that feels safe, calm, and entirely yours.

Building Your Daily Joy Toolkit

Creating a toolkit for emotional well-being during menopause is like building a cozy sanctuary inside yourself, a place you can return to when hormonal waves feel overwhelming or the world seems a bit too much. From my years working with menopausal women and from my own messy midlife experience, I've learned that joy isn't just a luxury, it's essential. It's healing. It's medicine for our changing bodies, minds, and spirits.

I learned this lesson the hard way myself. After pushing myself to the edge and believing, like many of us do, that I was invincible, finally listening to my body's screams of "Stop!" made me wonder if I'd ever feel like myself again. I was disconnected and extraordinarily tired in a way no nap could fix. But then, small glimpses of light began to emerge in slow, tiny, unexpected moments.

My little Australian terrier, Baxter, and my beautiful old Labrador, Stan, became my sources of joy when I couldn't find it anywhere else. They would chase each other around the yard like crazy. Sometimes, my grumpy British Blue cat would join in, and on especially funny days, a rogue mouse would join the chaos (don't worry; no mice were harmed;

the cat just liked the thrill). Amid all the madness, I'd find myself laughing. Truly laughing. And it felt like I was breathing for the first time in weeks.

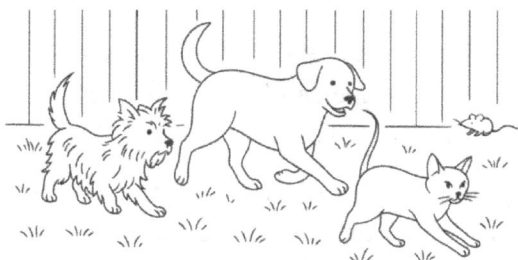

Those tiny moments became my lifeline. They felt natural and genuine. They reminded me that joy isn't always found in the big moments. Sometimes, it's in a wagging tail, a silly game of chase, or a quiet cup of tea in the sun where, just for a second, you feel at peace.

So, I started collecting those moments, noticing them, and leaning into them. Bit by bit, I built a Joy Toolkit: small daily rituals and simple pleasures that anchored me and reminded me of who I really was beneath the fatigue and fog. Now, I teach my clients to do the same, because you can't just think your way out of exhaustion. But you can definitely feel your way toward joy with one dog snuggle, sock-slip shuffle, or spontaneous giggle fit at a time.

Simple Daily Practices

That's where my Joy Toolkit started. It came from a place of desperation. I just wanted to feel something light again, something that reminded me I was still present, still myself.

Over time, I added small but meaningful practices that kept me grounded, even on the toughest days. Below, you'll find the core elements that helped me rebuild from the inside out: think of them as gentle suggestions rather than a checklist. Try what resonates with you, skip what doesn't. Your joy toolkit is yours to create.

Mindful Moments

Carve out small moments of stillness in your day. This might mean actually tasting your morning tea, feeling the warmth of the mug in your hands, or taking three slow breaths before walking into a busy room. For me, it's my early morning ritual: sitting quietly in my lush backyard while the world is still waking, with detox tea in hand. My little Aussie terrier, Baxter, instinctively knows this is our sacred time together. He always jumps onto my lap, tail wagging, as if to say, "It's you and me, Mom. What's the plan?"

Nature Connection

Even just five minutes outside can work wonders for your nervous system. Tune into your senses: see, hear, smell, touch, taste. Watch the clouds, smell your herbs, and stand barefoot on the grass. It just has to feel real. I've found that growing and eating from my own garden brings me genuine, grounded joy. And yes, gifting a homegrown cucumber to a friend feels oddly satisfying. It's like saying, "Here's a crunchy little miracle I raised myself."

Movement for Joy

Let go of the rules and move in a way that feels good: twirl in your garden, wiggle your hips while brushing your teeth, stretch like a sleepy cat. In my studio sessions, I often blend tai-chi-inspired flow with intuitive movement. We breathe into physically and emotionally tight spots and invite softness.

So often in life, we move in straight lines, forgetting that bodies, like feelings, need space to twist, sway, spiral, and stretch. Just watch your fur baby in the morning; what's the first thing they do? They stretch.

Creative Expression

Doodle. Paint. Sing badly in the shower. Make a joyful mess. Let go of the idea that you need to get it "right." This is your space to color outside the lines, use glitter for no reason, or write a poem no one else will ever read. Let it be imperfect, utterly ridiculous, and perfectly freeing. Because creativity isn't about outcomes at all; it's about feeling alive. And midlife is the perfect time to rediscover that feeling. If anyone dares to ask, "What on earth is she doing now?" just smile, grab your paintbrush or dance shoes, and say, "I'm building my joy toolkit. And no, I haven't gone mad; I've finally come back to myself."

Joy is your lifeline. Even just a few moments a day can begin to lift the emotional fog of menopause. These small, soulful rituals focus on presence. They'll help you vibrantly express the woman you are in the midst of it.

Joy Journal Prompt

What are the small moments that bring you joy when everything else feels overwhelming? Think of the things that make you smile effortlessly. The grounding, silly, soulful, or sensory moments that remind you that you're still here. Still you. Maybe it's the quiet hum of the house before anyone else wakes up. The way your dog greets you like a celebrity at the door. A stranger's smile that feels like it was meant just for you. Or the sudden sparkle of a rainbow when you weren't even looking for one.

Write them all down, or sketch them out if that feels right, without reservation. Let them come to life on the page. These are your breadcrumbs back to your happiness and the foundation of your personal Joy Toolkit. Over time, they'll guide you to your daily practice of gratitude, a way to honor the small, shining sparks that lift you up. With consistency, this practice blossoms into a daily ritual that gently reconnects you with what feels good, shines a light on what truly matters, and reminds you of all that's already working in your life.

Let me gently remind you that the magic lies in showing up for yourself, even in small ways. A laugh, a walk, a deep breath: they all matter. Small joys are nourishment for your nervous system. They help build emotional resilience, lighting the path through the fog and staying with you for life.

Rewrite the Script

When you change your story from "I'm broken" to "I'm becoming," the whole world opens up to you again. Joy begins to rise. Confidence stirs. Energy follows your curiosity. You're not behind. You're on the edge of something beautifully new. That's because the biggest obstacle to creativity isn't time or talent. It's the story you whisper to yourself. It could be: "I'm not creative," or "I'm too old to start." Perhaps it's even, "It's too late." But those aren't truths; they're just tired old scripts. And here's the good news: You can rewrite them. Try saying, "I'm learning how to light myself up again." You could also go with, "Now is exactly the right time." Because joy lives in the small, brave act of beginning.

A No-Rules Paint Session

Need a gentle, joyful way back to your creative center?

You could try this:

- Grab a big sheet of paper

- Choose three to five bold acrylic colors

- Put on your favorite playlist, the one that makes your hips sway

- Hit *play* ... and paint like no one's watching.

There's no pressure. Use whatever feels right: your hands, your feet, a sponge, a stick. In fact, use anything but a brush if you want to break the rules. Smear. Splatter. Layer. Let it be messy and magnificent. This kind of unfiltered expression bypasses perfectionism and taps into the freedom your inner child still craves. Let that playful inner child that used to be there come out and play. Your wild, curious girl is still here. Let her dance.

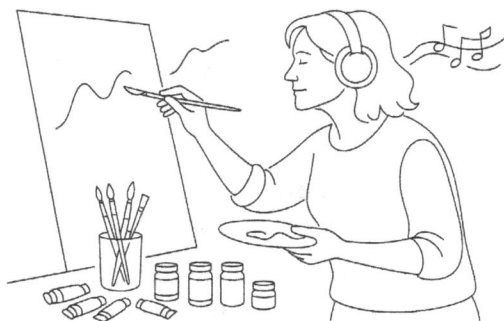

Your Mojo is Evolving

This is the start of a new relationship, with your energy, your story, your joy, and your spark. I'll never forget when Lisa, a longtime Pilates client, walked into the studio glowing. Not from a new serum or holiday, but from something deeper. She looked at me and said, "I finally get it. This isn't about fixing myself. It's about growing into who I'm meant to become." Yes! That's it. Midlife isn't a crisis; it's a creative portal. Your body is whispering and sometimes shouting, *"Let's do things differently now."* Do them richer. Softer. More soulful.

Through these pages, I hope you've not only reconnected with your energy but also with yourself. The wise, vibrant, capable woman who's been there all along, even beneath the fatigue, the people-pleasing, the fog. Yes, she's still here, and oh, she's magnificent!

Of course, there will still be low-energy days. Hormonal chaos. Moments when your motivation disappears. That's okay. On those days, show up gently. Start small, stretch your body, press *play* on your favorite tunes, drink a big glass of water with lemon, toss together a rainbow-bright salad, laugh at something silly, close your eyes for a nap, or let your body follow the music. It just has to be kind. And maybe, just maybe, we could learn to take life a little less seriously.

What happened to that girl who used to belly laugh out loud, dance wildly when the mood struck, no hesitation, no apology? She's just been waiting for permission to come back out and play.

Whatever fuels your fire and rekindles your spark, follow that. A quiet moment, a song, a stretch, a connection: let it be what makes your soul sing as you gradually reconnect with your body and spirit. And when you doubt yourself, because we all do, remember you've already overcome so much in your lifetime. You've grown in ways that prove your strength.

Midlife isn't something to fix; it's something to honor because growing older is a privilege. This is your moment to check in with how you're feeling physically, emotionally, and mentally, and to gently redesign life so it fits who you are now. You don't need a dramatic reset; you need a clear, kind next step.

Remember, your energy and joy aren't gone; they're just waiting for you to notice them again. One walk, one paint stroke, one song at a time. That's how you rebuild your spark, and that's how midlife becomes your most radiant chapter yet.

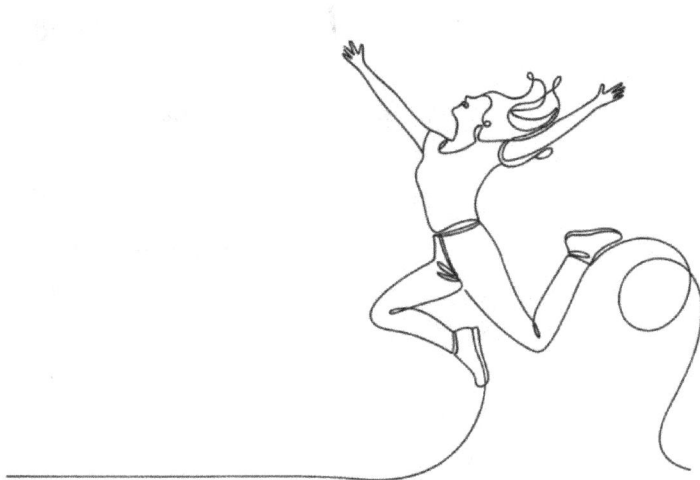

CHAPTER 18

Your Midlife Renaissance

"Change your story, change your life. Divorce the story of limitation and marry the story of truth and everything changes."

– TONY ROBBINS

Change Your Story

If there's one person whose work truly lit a spark and set me on a new path, it's Tony Robbins. I'm a proud Master graduate of all his main live courses, and I can honestly say his teachings helped me change how I was living and who I thought I had to be.

I first heard about Tony from my dear friend, Juliet. She was going through a tough time and decided to fly overseas for one of his big events in Hawaii. I dropped her off at the airport, and when I picked her up ten days later, I didn't recognize the woman who came back. She was glowing. Her eyes sparkled. It was like her soul had stepped forward. I looked at her and said, "I don't know what just happened, but I want what you're having. Sign me up."

Back then, I was running a large, male-dominated photography business. This was thirty years ago, when you had to be tough to be taken seriously as a woman in that world. I wore a black suit every day. I didn't own a single dress or any color in my wardrobe. I had long, black, plaited African braids. I drove a black convertible and had a fierce-looking black Rottweiler named Robaryn, although he had the temperament of a

Labrador. Everything about me said "power." And, on the outside, I looked like I had it all together.

Then came Tony. Through his teachings, I reclaimed my feminine power.

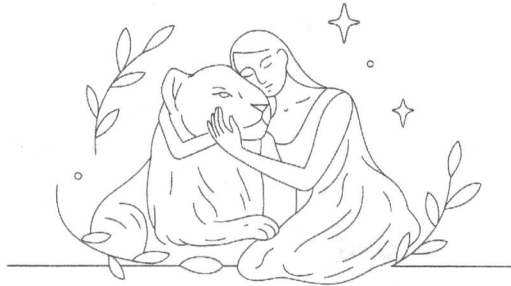

One moment I'll never forget is standing in what Tony would call "Peak State," barefoot at night, staring down a fifty-foot fire walk in Hawaii. Real hot coals. Real heat. No tricks. And somehow, I walked across it barefoot, steady, and completely unburned. That moment wasn't just about bravado or hype. It was about awakening something ancient within me: a knowing, a remembering. I learned that, if I could walk over fire, I could survive anything. That fear didn't get to be the driver anymore.

Courage, I discovered, isn't about feeling fearless. It's about taking a deep breath, rolling your shoulders back, and stepping forward anyway. That I could change my life, starting right then and there, in a heartbeat.

That night in Hawaii lit something inside me. And it wasn't just adrenaline or "rah-rah" motivation. It was rewiring.

Science now shows that the stories we tell ourselves literally shape our brains. When you repeat a thought, "I'm not good enough," or "I'm too old to change," it strengthens neural pathways, making that belief feel true. But when you tell yourself something different: "I am strong and resilient," "I am open to learning and growing," "I get to choose differently," your brain begins to make new connections. This is called neuroplasticity, and it's transformative stuff.

In midlife, when hormones, roles, and identities are shifting, story becomes more than words. It becomes a map. Change the story, and you change the route your nervous system follows. Instead of spiraling into fear or fatigue, or the dreaded "what now?" your body and mind start practicing courage, calm, and curiosity.

That's why this work matters so much. It's not about pretending everything is perfect or chanting affirmations you don't believe. It's about practicing a new narrative until it becomes your lived truth. The story you tell yourself every day isn't just background noise; it's your life's soundtrack. So, you might as well make it a song worth dancing to.

Newness and Curiosity

After that experience, everything changed. I abandoned the black masculine suits. I let go of the version of myself I thought success had required. My wardrobe went from fifty shades of black to an explosion of color, and honestly, my mood followed suit. I now embrace softness and femininity as strength and power. I've become bold in a different way, one that feels more like me than anything else ever has. Because here's what I've learned: You don't have to shrink to fit in. And you definitely don't have to dress like a corporate ninja to be taken seriously. What sets you apart is your superpower, your quirks, your voice, your uniqueness, your lived wisdom. Your true power isn't something to perform; it's already in you, waiting for your soul to take off its invisibility cloak and shine.

Too often, we live in fear, afraid of failing or of not being enough. At midlife, this fear can feel louder, as though life has reached a standstill. The children have grown and left home, the roles of mother, cook, housekeeper, and partner may no longer define the shape of each day, and for many of us, the loss of a parent leaves us without a mentor to lean on. Yet, this is also where the turning point lies.

Nelson Mandela said, "I learned that courage was not the absence of fear, but the triumph over it." Stepping into the unknown at this stage of life can be deeply freeing. It's like pressing "refresh" on a long-forgotten app: you're still you, but with fewer bugs and better boundaries. It is a chance to be adventurous, courageous, and curious, to discover who you truly are without the constraints of past identities. Midlife becomes less about what you have lost and more about what you are finally free to find.

It is easy to feel lost, uncertain of who you are or where you belong. Yet, this season can also be a doorway into something new. When you face the fear and step forward anyway, you begin to build a muscle of courage and resilience. Midlife becomes a chance to rediscover yourself, to move beyond old identities and explore what truly brings you alive. It's like trying on a new version of yourself. It can feel freeing, adventurous, and exciting, like setting out on a new path where the destination is not yet known but full of possibility.

I believe that spark was always within me. I was the girl from little old New Zealand who earned a scholarship to study photography in New York in her twenties and received numerous international awards for my creativity. Somewhere along the way, I got too busy being sensible. Like so many of us do, I just needed permission to stop hiding it.

What has guided me through every reinvention is this truth: "The greatest obstacle between you and the life you desire is the story you've come to believe about yourself." When you shift that story, something magical happens, and midlife is the perfect moment to do just that. It's your cue to step into the spotlight, sequins optional, and take center stage in your next chapter.

Reframing Midlife

Of course, the transition through menopause can feel like an ending. But, more often, it's the start of something much more powerful. Thriving through it transforms you, like a butterfly emerging from the chrysalis, just a bit sweatier. This phase can ignite creative passion and a deep reconnection to your purpose.

As Cher once said, "All of us invent ourselves. Some of us have more imagination than others." Midlife is your invitation to become your own creative project. It's a time to imagine boldly, to play with possibility, and to give yourself permission to reinvent who you are becoming.

I experienced that shift firsthand. One day, after my turning point, I sat quietly in the garden. I was watching the seasons change when I heard a whisper from deep inside, "What if this is the beginning, not the end?" It wasn't a dramatic Hollywood moment. No thunderbolt or celestial light show. Just a quiet knowing that something new was calling. From that stillness, I started to reimagine what my next chapter could look like. It didn't begin with goals; it started with truth. It starts with getting honest, slowing down, listening carefully, and giving yourself permission to dream again, but this time, on your terms, with midlife wisdom, clarity, and unapologetic vision.

Before we start imagining your dream future, we need to begin with what's real. The unfiltered version. Many women are in full-on survival mode: tired, burned-out, overwhelmed, and laser-focused on fixing their symptoms. They want to know how to beat the hot flashes, brain fog, and insomnia now! I get it. These are no small things. But menopause isn't something we're meant to just endure and fight through. It's not a storm to be weathered. It's something we evolve through.

Jennifer came to me in exactly that exhausted, empty state. She was doing everything she could to manage the symptoms, but when I gently asked her what she actually wanted from this next chapter, she just blinked. It hadn't occurred to her that she was allowed to want more than symptom relief, that thriving was even an option, not just surviving with an ice pack and herbal tea.

So, we started small. I asked her, "What does thriving look like for you?" The truth is, we don't always begin considering the future until something, or someone, wakes us up. For me, it happened when I saw loved ones start to age. Watching my dad lose his independence and seeing friends' parents decline into dementia was my reality check. It hit me like a whispered reminder: "Life is short, but it's not over." It made me ask myself, "How do I want to be at eighty, and at ninety? What kind of life do I want to be living? And what choices am I making now to get me there?"

Redesigning Your Second Act

We're not here to just bounce back. We're here to move forward with clarity, wisdom, and unapologetic self-worth. Your Second Act is about coming home to yourself, about redesigning your life to reflect who you truly are now.

Maybe your vision for your Second Act includes feeling strong and energized again. Maybe it's about doing work that lights you up, creating a home that reflects your soul, or finally letting go of roles and relationships that no longer serve you.

Maybe it's about exploring that "crazy" dream you buried years ago. Reclaiming your creativity. Rediscovering your sensuality. Or simply learning to be still. Whatever it is, this is more than just the next chapter; it's a whole new book. And you are the author now.

Creating your Second Act Vision can be an ongoing work in progress. In fact, some of the most meaningful shifts I've seen start in the quietest moments: on the back porch with a cup of tea, during a nature walk, or scribbled on a napkin at a dinner party with friends. They also continue to unfold naturally, without striving to achieve anything specific. After guiding many women through this stage and my own self-discovery, I've noticed certain patterns that help light the way forward.

Many of us have spent decades putting others first: caregivers, achievers, the reliable ones. Our workplaces, bosses, workloads, stress, and tendency to overcommit have shaped how we show up. We made choices based on what was expected or convenient for everyone else. But now? Now it's your season to switch from autopilot to intentional living. This is your season to turn inward.

Ask yourself, gently and honestly, "What do I want?" and "What actually lights me up these days?" Let go of the "shoulds" and listen for the quiet voice of who you are now.

Self-discovery isn't reinvention. It's remembering. It's coming home to what feels true to you and trusting that you're allowed to change. Get curious and let the answers surprise you. Because sometimes the thing that lights you up isn't a grand new goal. It's simply getting your sparkle back, one small joy at a time.

Give yourself permission to dream. Let go of outdated roles and inherited expectations. Give yourself full permission to imagine something different and bold that fits you now. And if anyone rolls their eyes or says, "She's lost the plot," you can smile and reply, "Actually, I'm writing a better one."

Surround yourself with people who reflect your strength back to you. Whether it's your Pilates group, your book club, or a circle of wise women, find your people. Connection is grounding, healing, and reminds you that we're never walking this road alone.

This is about gently expanding what's possible while staying deeply attuned to what your body, heart, and soul need right now. Think of it as planting seeds for your future while nourishing your present.

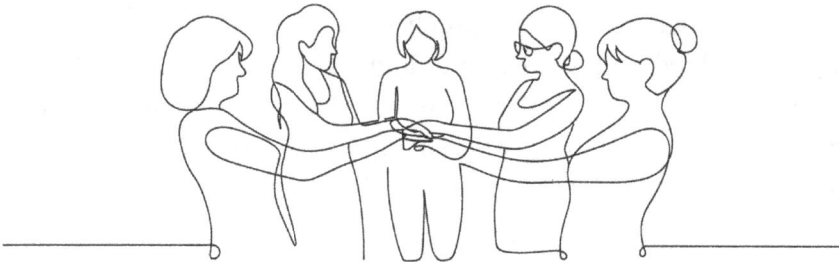

Visioning Practices

One practice I return to again and again is my Life Journal. It's a messy mix of thoughts, highlighters, doodles, sticky notes, and soul whispers. It's not Instagram pretty, but it's real, part dream diary, part brain dump, and part therapy session. I think of it as my compass: If you don't set a destination, you end up circling the block, unsure where you're heading. But when you put things on paper, it's like opening a map: the route appears, turn by turn.

It's a creative space to dream, reflect, and reimagine. If you have a partner, you might each keep your own journals, then share your visions.

It can be revealing, fun, and deeply connecting. You might even discover you've both been dreaming of the same beach house or entirely different continents. Either way, it starts a great conversation.

Your journal is your sandbox, a space to ask big questions and entertain bold ideas:

- What would you do if you couldn't fail?

- What makes you lose track of time (in the best way)?

- What wisdom have you earned that the world needs to hear?

- What have you never done that you want to do? Choose something that makes your heart sing, perhaps something as adventurous as walking the Camino de Santiago.

Something magical happens when pen meets paper. The slower pace quiets the noise, sparks creativity, and lets ideas flow in ways a keyboard rarely can. So, grab some writing paper, find a quiet space, pour a cup of tea, and let your thoughts wander. And if you don't finish in one sitting, that's perfectly fine; come back to it later.

The point is simply to let your dreams flow. This space is just for you.

I've kept a Life Journal for twenty years, and looking back amazes me. So many quiet dreams have found their way into reality. That's the gift of this practice. It gives you clarity, direction, and the courage to believe more is possible.

Once your vision starts to take shape, it's time to give it direction. Think of this as your Midlife GPS, a gentle guide that helps you find your way, one step at a time. Start by grounding yourself in the present: notice what's working, what brings joy, and what no longer fits. Reflect on the small wins, the choices that empowered you, and the lessons learned along the way.

From there, cast forward. Imagine what you'd love to do, create, or experience in the next year, and even ten. Choose a few goals that excite you and note *why* they matter. Then take one small action today, however simple: a call, a booking, a text, or a walk. Even a tiny step counts; momentum loves movement, no matter how small.

This isn't about perfection; it's about direction. When you dream, reflect, and take even the smallest step, you start to design a life that honors your energy, your body, and your joy.

Check in regularly, weekly, monthly, or yearly, in whatever rhythm that feels natural to you. What you focus on grows, so the more often you pause to reflect, the easier it becomes to see your progress. You'll be amazed how much shifts simply by paying attention.

This journey isn't about doing it all; it's about moving toward what matters most. When you plan it, you make it possible. When you act on it, you bring it to life. Because in the end, your vision isn't about becoming someone new; it's about remembering who you were always meant to be and giving her the steering wheel.

Vision Board

One of my favorite New Year's rituals is hosting a Vision Board Dinner Party. Each year, I invite a few friends over, set the table with good food and laughter, and cover the dining table with glue sticks, old magazines, and cardboard. It's less Martha Stewart, more organized chaos, but that's part of the charm. We sip wine and cut out images and words that represent our dreams. It's messy fun, often loud, and pure magic.

Last year, I placed a photo of the Amalfi Coast right in the middle of mine. At the time, it felt like a stretch. The kind of "maybe one day" dream you secretly hope the universe is eavesdropping on. But a few months later, I found myself standing in that same spot, glass of wine in hand, soaking in the sunset.

That's the thing about vision boards; they're equal parts imagination and gentle accountability. Once you've glued your dream down, it's amazing how life starts conspiring to meet you halfway. There's magic in having a vision, setting an intention, and finally saying "yes to myself."

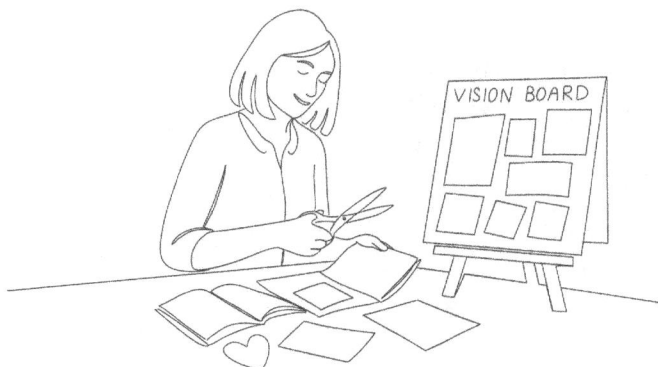

Your Own Renaissance

Think of this chapter of life as your own renaissance (without the corsets), a powerful creative rebirth. Only this time, there are no restrictions reserved for men only, no tight deadlines, and no one else dictating what it should look like.

There's just you, perhaps wearing your favorite Lululemon tights for freedom (and not just of movement), with a strong coffee at dawn, reinventing a wonderfully rich life on your terms. Like the great artists of the original Renaissance, you're carefully shaping a masterpiece, one inspired, soul-aligned step at a time.

Signing up for that retreat? Finally carving out space for rest? Dusting off an old dream and giving it one more go? All parts of the mosaic of who you are becoming, with more clarity, more courage, and a whole lot more color.

Pause and Reflect

As we near the end of the book, let's pause and revisit the five pillars we began with: mindset, nourishment, movement, connection, and purpose. Mindset is the quiet turn from forcing to listening, curiosity over criticism. Nutrition calms the body with simple, protein-forward plates and plenty of color so energy feels even instead of spiky. Movement becomes a dialogue to tune in, not a drill; some days you lift, other days you trade the plan for a gentle Pilates flow, a walk with a friend, or slow, focused stretching, and yes, planned rest days absolutely count.

Connection is your soft landing: shared laughter, a quick walk, a text, the comfort of being understood. Purpose is your North Star, the steady why behind your choices. Start tiny today: a reframed thought, a nourishing plate, ten minutes that match your energy, a message to someone you love, or one true line in your Life Journal. That's how it all weaves together: gentle daily rhythms, a body you can trust, and a life that feels beautifully, unapologetically yours.

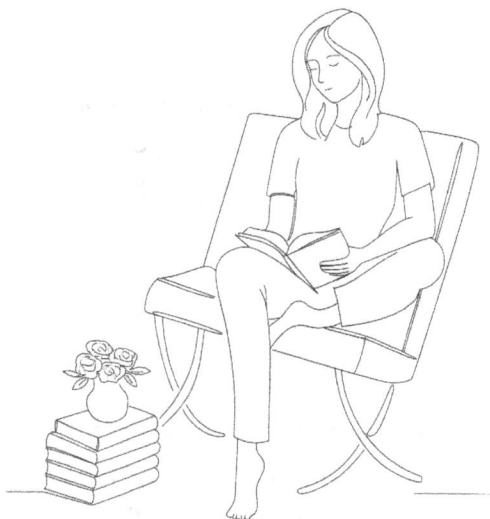

CHAPTER 19

Your Daily Balance Blueprint

"Routines get a bad rap because they can feel restrictive or confining at times. But when done correctly, routines are actually what free us!"

– ASHLEY NICOLE

Habits, Routines, and Rituals

Fifty caught me off guard. Not exactly like hitting a wall, though some days it felt like that, but more like missing a sharp turn in the road. It made me slow down and reevaluate my speed and direction. That pause made me look around and ask myself, "Wait… how did I get here?"

For me, that wake-up came wrapped in exhaustion so deep I could barely get through the day. I'd overwork and overexercise myself into burnout, going from constant motion to lying on the floor, unsure if I had the energy to lift a shopping bag or climb the stairs. Midlife didn't just ask me to do life differently; it asked me to be different. It was humbling. And in time, healing.

Habits, routines, and rituals may look ordinary on the surface, but they carry extraordinary power.

These anchors don't come from dramatic overhauls but from small, supportive practices, like tiny hinges that open big doors. A gentle scaffold you can lean on, especially when life feels chaotic or your hormones seem to have gone wild. Let's explore three essentials that are often lumped together but serve different roles: habits, routines, and rituals.

Habits That Stick

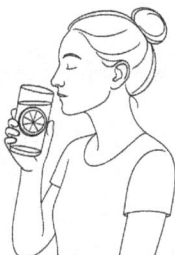

"Doing one thing by yourself, for yourself, that creates joy is such an important habit."

– JAY SHETTY

A habit is simply a behavior you repeat so often it becomes second nature. These are small actions your brain performs almost automatically, like brushing your teeth or reaching for your phone before your eyes are even open. They live in the basal ganglia, the efficiency center of your brain.

Habits save energy, which is exactly what your midlife brain craves. But here's the truth: Habits can work both ways. They can be nourishing, like a glass of lemon water in the morning, or quietly drain your vitality, like midnight fridge raids. And because your nervous system is more sensitive during menopause, the habits you choose to keep matter more than ever.

Routines for Your Nervous System

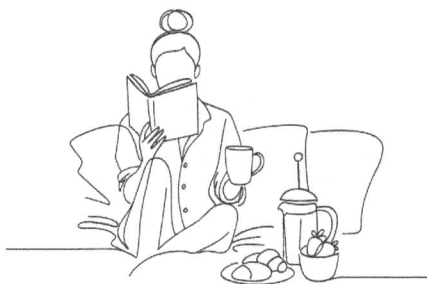

"Success is the sum of small efforts, repeated day in and day out."

– ROBERT COLLIER

If a habit is a single action, a routine is what happens when you string habits together with consistency. A routine is a pattern that creates rhythm and flow, and it provides a sense of safety. Where habits save energy, routines give structure. They turn scattered moments into something predictable, and predictability is soothing for your nervous system.

In the past, I resisted routines, feeling they were dull and too structured. Maybe that's the creative in me. But after hormonal chaos and full-blown burnout, routines became my anchor. They gave shape to the days and helped me listen more closely to what my body needed. I began to crave them. My morning routine of hydration, meditation, light movement, a few stretches, breakfast and five minutes of stillness with my fur baby became a daily anchor. On tough days, that routine is my soft landing, even if "stillness" looks more like sitting in sweatpants, resting more, sipping bone broth from a mug, and staring blankly into space.

Soulful Rituals

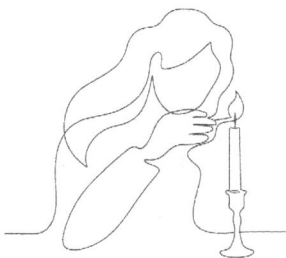

"Ritual is able to hold the long-discarded shards of our stories and make them whole again. It has the strength and elasticity to contain what we cannot contain on our own, what we cannot face in solitude."

– FRANCIS WELLER

Now, here's the one that gets me every time. If habits are actions and routines are patterns, rituals are meaning. Unlike habits or routines, rituals are sacred. They're infused with meaning and intention. Rituals slow you down, center you, and reconnect you with the self that lives beneath the to-do list.

Lighting a candle before journaling. Playing a certain song while getting dressed. Whispering a mantra as you step into your day. They're touchstones. Tiny moments of magic.

For me, it's picking up my dad's old, trusted hammer for DIY around the house. In those moments, I feel like I'm channeling his practical farmer's skills, and the job somehow turns out better than I expected. It's oddly nostalgic and deeply grounding. I glance at the photo of Dad on the fridge, and for a moment, he's with me again. That is a ritual.

Rituals don't have to be grand. They can be as small as a whispered thank you over morning tea, a walk at dusk with the dog, or flowers you buy for yourself every few weeks. Neuroscience backs this up: Rituals regulate the nervous system, soothe anxiety, and anchor us when life feels unsteady.

Habits automate the basics, routines create rhythm and flow and rituals add soul and meaning. Together, they form the gentle scaffolding that holds you when life feels chaotic or your hormones seem to have gone wild.

Before we step into each pillar of the Midlife Blueprint: mindset, movement, nourishment, rest, and connection, pause and notice your own patterns. Which habits carry you forward? Which routines give you flow? Which rituals bring you back to yourself? These are the anchors where lasting change begins.

Mindset: Your Inner Compass

Your thoughts shape the way you navigate midlife. A single thought can either drain your energy or open a door to possibility.

The way you start and end your day matters more than you think. Instead of reaching for your phone first thing, try giving yourself ten quiet minutes to breathe and settle your mind. You'll be amazed how much better the day feels when you don't start it by scrolling through someone else's highlight reel. That small act of stillness sets the tone for how you want to feel and show up.

At the other end of the day, create a small ritual to switch off from work. A warm shower can wash away the weight of the day, and changing into fresh clothes signals to your body that it's time to rest. You might finish by writing a few lines of gratitude in your journal. Sometimes it's something big, and sometimes it's as small as a client's kind message or the fact that you resisted replying to emails after nine p.m. (a true midlife superpower). These moments build a quiet bond with yourself, reminding you that you're doing better than you think.

Throughout the day, check in with the tone of your self-talk. Do you speak to yourself with kindness or criticism? When you make a mistake, return to a phrase that steadies you: "I am learning. I am growing. I am enough." That simple habit of gentle self-talk becomes a ritual of resilience and deepens your bond with your own wellbeing.

Other rituals help you soften. Lighting a candle and listening to some soft tunes. Placing a hand on your heart when anxiety rises. Taking three conscious deep belly breaths before walking into a meeting or class. And perhaps the most powerful one of all: saying no when you feel yourself about to overcommit. Each of these small acts is sacred. They whisper to my nervous system, "It is safe to pause. It is safe to soften."

The science is clear: Mindset rituals and routines don't just shift your mood; they rewire your brain. Repeated practices of calm, gratitude, and self-compassion strengthen neural pathways, reduce cortisol, and improve resilience. For women in midlife, this means a steadier nervous system, more balanced hormones, and greater emotional clarity.

Even as a coach, just like many of you, I still catch myself in old patterns of pushing, proving, or people-pleasing. The structure makes consistency possible. The rituals make it meaningful.

Before you set your mindset for today, pause and ask, "What do I need most right now: clarity, calm, courage, or kindness?" Then go give yourself exactly that, without guilt, and preferably with good music and a strong cup of tea.

Nourishment That Grounds You

Food is how you steady your hormones and energy. It's not about getting everything right but about creating rhythms that support balance, not chaos. When you eat in a way that feels nourishing and consistent, your body learns to trust you again and stops thinking it needs to survive on caffeine and willpower.

Many women find that gentle structure brings calm to their energy and hormones. You might experiment with eating windows that suit your lifestyle, perhaps a midmorning breakfast, an afternoon meal, and an early dinner to allow a natural overnight fast. What matters most is making those meals count with protein-rich, nutrient-dense, colorful meals that keep you feeling grounded and satisfied.

Choose one day each week to anchor your habits. Sundays, for example, can be your reset: shop for staples and prepare a few nourishing basics so the fridge is ready for the week ahead. Hummus, coconut yogurt, eggs, salmon, chopped veggies, and a jar of nuts are simple staples that make it easy to stay on track. Without that structure, hunger and convenience take over, and that's when the toast and peanut butter tends to make its grand return.

Then come the rituals. Sit down to eat whenever possible, ideally without screens or distractions. Step outside if you can. Savor each mouthful and notice the colors, textures, and smells. Between meals, hydrate well by filling your stainless-steel bottles each morning with water or herbal teas so you're prepared for the day. Bonus: carrying them around makes you feel slightly virtuous before you've even taken a sip.

That pause, that attention, transforms food from fuel into nourishment. It becomes a way of grounding myself, of reminding my body that it is safe, cared for, and worthy of good things.

Nutrition is a cornerstone of resilience in midlife, supporting hormone balance, energy, and clarity. When you nourish well, you steady everything else.

Movement That Works

Movement is one of the most important anchors in midlife. It steadies your energy, lifts your mood, and clears your mind enough to remember what you came into the room for. Creating a rhythm that fits real life.

Think of it as your personal framework: perhaps strength training three times a week, walking in nature on alternate days, and leaving room for Pilates, stretching, or a long hill walk with a friend on the weekend. Those walks aren't just about fitness; they're therapy in sneakers, full of laughter, connection, and catching up on each other's latest "midlife discoveries." Rest days count, too, giving your body time to recharge and respond. Without that structure, the "I'll start tomorrow" trap wins far too easily.

Then come the rituals. Hydrating well, refueling with a protein-rich meal within the hour, and celebrating the post-workout glow instead of rushing to the next thing. These small, sacred anchors support recovery, hydration, and muscle strength. Movement becomes more than a workout; it becomes a way to bond with your body, your friends, and your sense of self.

Life has a way of crowding out exercise, especially for women juggling work, home, and the endless to-do list. The structure makes consistency possible. The rituals make it meaningful.

Before you move today, pause and ask, "How do I want to feel when I finish? Strong? Calm? Flexible? Uplifted?" Then choose accordingly. Some days it might be heavy weights, other days a dog walk, Pilates, or simply stretching out the day's tension while dinner cooks. It all counts.

Research confirms what many of us feel in our bones: Regular movement is a cornerstone of midlife health. It improves muscle mass, protects bone density, balances blood sugar, and reduces the risk of heart disease. It also lowers cortisol and boosts mood, giving both body and mind resilience. It's the ultimate energy reset and let's face it, nothing beats the satisfaction of knowing you kept a promise to yourself.

Rest Matters More

Sleep is how you restore your body, mind, and sanity. It's not a luxury or a sign of weakness; it's one of your greatest tools for balance. Think of rest as your invisible workout: The time when your body repairs, your hormones reset, and your brain quietly files away the day's chaos.

Creating a calm evening rhythm helps your body know what's coming. Eat dinner early, dim the lights, and trade screens for something soothing, like a warm shower, a cup of tea, or a few slow breaths before bed. Keeping your bedtime and wake-up time roughly the same each day (yes, even on weekends) helps your body clock stay on track.

Add small rituals that feel like comfort. Light a candle, stretch on the floor, or write down three small things that went right today. Lavender spray on the pillow helps, but so does laughter. Try a feel-good movie or a chat with a friend who makes you laugh until you snort. Each of these simple acts whispers to your nervous system, "It's safe to rest."

Rest days matter, too. They're not wasted time; they're your repair time. Think of them as your body's way of saying thank you for showing up day after day.

Consistent sleep routines and gentle rituals help your body shift from "go" to "restore." For women in midlife, that's a real gift. Quality sleep supports hormone balance, reduces cortisol, regulates appetite, and brings back that grounded, clear feeling that makes life flow a little easier.

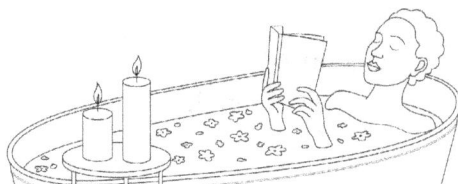

Connection and Joy

Joy is medicine. Each week, pause to ask yourself, "What brought me joy? What moments made me laugh, light up, and feel like myself again?" These tiny sparks, scattered through ordinary days, are not frivolous extras. They are fuel for your spirit.

Joy often hides in simple rituals. Maybe it's the way your dog greets you like you've returned from a six-month expedition every single morning, or that first quiet coffee in the sun before the world wakes up. Fresh flowers on the kitchen table, a walk with a friend who makes you laugh, or a message to check in on someone who's been on your mind. None of it needs to be grand. It just needs to be genuine.

And then there's play. Yes, actual play. The kind that involves grass stains, laughter, or singing off-key in the car with the windows down. Joy expands when you let yourself be a little silly again. If you can, plan something to look forward to. A dinner with friends, a weekend away, or your own version of the "Fabulous 50s Crew" adventure that gets booked before the last one even ends.

These rituals are intentional anchors of happiness. Midlife can so easily get swallowed by roles and responsibilities, yet rituals of joy remind us that we are not just caretakers, partners, or professionals. We are women who laugh, who play, who create, love, and sometimes snort at our own jokes.

Research shows that joy and laughter are not just luxuries; they lower cortisol, boost immunity, and strengthen resilience. Even small moments of joy act like medicine for the nervous system, reminding your body that it's safe to relax, to connect, and to live with a little more lightness. Joy isn't frivolous; it's fuel for healing and vitality.

Small Shifts, Big Change

When it comes to supporting hormonal health during menopause, grand plans are nice, but it's the small, consistent actions that actually shift the dial.

One of my clients, Kate, came to me with five meditation apps, stacks of wellness books, and a laminated meal plan she could never stick to. She was burning herself out doing "all the right things." So, we started with just one stacked habit: three deep breaths every time she turned on her computer. That was it. No scented mist. No mountaintop getaway. Just presence.

When that stuck, we added another: a desk stretch after each call and a water bottle within reach. Weeks later, her shoulders finally started to unclench and she laughed, "I think my neck just forgave me."

That's how habit stacking works. They're like acupuncture for your day: tiny points of intention that reset your whole system. They're gentle, doable, and work by linking a new habit to something you already do.

When I finish my shower, I do a thirty-second cool rinse.

When I put on deodorant, I take my supplements.

When I plan the week on Sunday, I book one friend walk and a rest day.

When I start cooking, I balance on one leg for thirty seconds.

When it's an hour to bedtime, I make herbal tea and silence notifications.

Why does this work? Because your brain loves anchors. One cue leads to the next until the sequence runs on autopilot. That's a gift in midlife, when energy and motivation can ebb and flow more than we'd like to admit.

Start gently. One anchor. One habit. Then build. Over time, these layers create real rhythm and resilience.

Habits automate the basics, routines create flow, and rituals add soul. Together, they become anchors when the ground feels unsteady. But underneath them all lies something deeper: purpose. Purpose is what makes your habits worth repeating, your routines worth keeping, and your rituals worth cherishing.

Purpose: The Thread That Weaves It Together

"The two most important days in your life are the day you are born and the day you discover why."

– MARK TWAIN

These words remind us that purpose isn't just a lofty idea; it's the heartbeat of a meaningful life.

At midlife, purpose rarely arrives as a thunderclap or a carved-in-stone mission. It's more likely to sneak up on you while you're watering the plants, chatting with a friend, or halfway through your morning coffee. It is the heartbeat beneath your habits, the steady why that gives meaning to all the small, sometimes repetitive acts of care you practice each day.

Psychologists sometimes describe meaning in life as a three-legged stool: coherence, significance, and purpose. Coherence helps to make sense of your story and connects where you've been with where you are now. Significance reminds you that you matter and that you make a difference. And purpose gives you a reason to get up in the morning that doesn't involve feeding the dog or finding your reading glasses.

When midlife shakes the ground beneath us, through changing hormones, shifting family roles, or career shifts, it can make the stool wobble. But rather than calling it a "midlife crisis," think of it as a cosmic furniture adjustment. A crossroads, and chance to steady yourself and ask, "Am I still living in alignment with what matters most?"

This is your Balance Blueprint. Think of it as five strong pillars that hold you steady:

- Mindset gives you clarity and shapes how you see yourself.

- Nourishment steadies your energy and hormones.

- Movement builds your strength and resilience.

- Rest restores your body and mind.

- Connection softens life's edges and fills you with meaning.

Purpose is the thread that weaves them all together. It is what reminds you why you bother to choose protein at lunch, lace up your sneakers, turn your phone on "do not disturb" at night, or sit quietly and exhale in peace with a cup of tea when everyone else is doom-scrolling.

Your purpose may be raising strong daughters, mentoring others, creating something wildly imperfect, finally starting that herb garden you've been talking about for five years. It doesn't have to be grand to matter; it only needs to feel true to you.

Purpose can live in many places. It might be the way you show up for your family with an open heart, as a supportive mother or loving partner, offering stability and love in the middle of change. It might be the courage to finally share your creative work, even if it is only with yourself. It might be nurturing something that grows slowly, like a friendship, a community group, or a patch of soil in your backyard. For some, purpose is found in service, supporting someone who needs encouragement, passing on hard-earned wisdom, or making space for someone else's voice to be heard.

What gives life meaning is rarely flashy. It is often woven into the ordinary: the meals you prepare with care, the conversations you linger in, the rituals that tether you to memory and belonging. Purpose can evolve, too. What lit you up in your thirties may shift in your fifties, and that is part of the beauty. In my twenties, I thought Pilates was too slow for my adrenaline-fueled workouts. Now I crave it, not only because I understand how good it is for my body, but because I can feel the difference in my flexibility and core strength. Sharing that has become one of my greatest gifts. My purpose breathes and grows with me.

Science now shows what many of us feel intuitively: People with a sense of purpose live longer, healthier lives. Purpose steadies our minds, strengthens our bodies, and keeps us curious. It improves not only health markers, like cognition, grip strength, and longevity, but also the quality of our everyday lives. Purpose isn't only about having something to live for. It's about having something that keeps us truly alive.

I have met so many women who discovered new purpose in this season. Amanda left a high-powered executive role to start a community garden and become a mentor, passing her skills to the next generation. Once she adjusted to life without an overflowing inbox, she found her health, energy, and joy grew when she aligned her life with deeper values. That is the gift of midlife: It offers the chance to reevaluate, to shed what no longer fits, and to build again on a foundation of what truly matters.

The key is to notice. Notice what makes your heart soften, when time disappears, and when you feel most fully yourself. The hours you lose in the garden until you finally look up, dirty-handed and deeply satisfied. The laughter that lingers long after a meal with friends. Those are the breadcrumbs. The moments when time disappears and you feel most alive. Follow them, and you begin to live not from obligation but from alignment.

Every nourishing meal says, "My energy matters." Every walk, stretch, or weight lifted tells your body, "I'm strong enough for what's next." Every laugh, cuddle, or act of kindness whispers, "This is the kind of woman I choose to be." And here is the beautiful truth: Purpose is not a destination. It is a rhythm lived in ordinary choices repeated with intention. It is in how you begin, how you pause, and how you close your day.

When you live with purpose, even the smallest act, such as a deep breath, a shared laugh, or a plate of colorful food, becomes sacred. And that is the true blueprint for a life that feels whole, joyful, and beautifully your own. That is the invitation of midlife: to live not smaller, but truer, with purpose as your guide and plenty of laughter along the way.

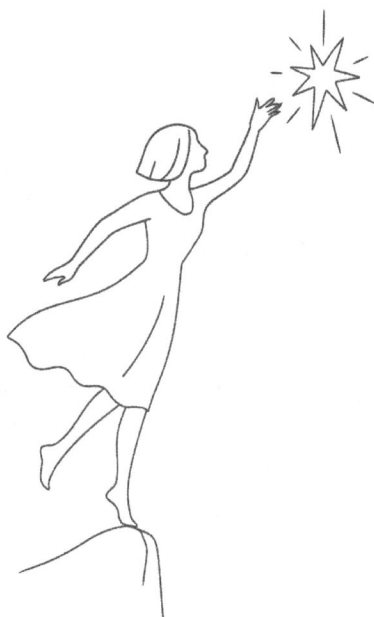

Conclusion

"The purpose of life, after all, is to live it, to taste
experience to the utmost, to reach out eagerly and without
fear for newer and richer experience"

– ELEANOR ROOSEVELT.

Your Radiant Years: Your Second Act

As we finish this journey together, I want to share one essential truth: This is only the beginning. Midlife can hit like a storm, exhausting and confusing. I know that place well. It made me question everything: how I was living, what I was prioritizing, and who I wanted to become. My crisis became the turning point for change. I took better care of myself in a new way. I started to rediscover joy, genuine joy, the kind that's personal and powerful. That's what I hope this book has given you: inspiration to heal, dream, and rise. To create your next chapter on your own terms and build a life full of purpose, vitality, and deep, unapologetic joy.

We've been told for too long that menopause is a decline, a slow fade, but it's not. It's an awakening. A fierce and beautiful transition into a chapter where your wisdom deepens, your voice grows stronger, and your soul becomes louder. One of my clients said it perfectly, "This isn't about fixing what's broken. It's about becoming who I was always meant to be." That shift, from viewing ourselves as problems to be fixed to seeing ourselves as people still growing and evolving, changes everything.

When I look around, I see two paths emerging in midlife and beyond. Some people shrink, give up. Their days become smaller, and their spark fades. But others expand. They explore. They become more vibrant than ever before. The difference lies in purpose, joy, connection, movement, and curiosity.

I've long been intrigued by the research on Blue Zones, those rare areas around the world where people live vibrantly into their nineties and even beyond. While genetics contribute to longevity, lifestyle often has a much bigger influence. Longevity is not just about adding years to your life; it is about adding life to your years. It is not enough to reach a certain age. What matters is living well, in good health, so you can keep doing the things you love, staying active, engaged, and connected.

In these communities, rates of chronic disease are surprisingly low. What's their secret? It's not a miracle supplement or an elite gym membership. It's their daily habits. They move naturally: walking, gardening, climbing hills. They eat mostly plant-based foods: seasonal vegetables, legumes, whole grains, and nuts, with small amounts of local fish. They follow the 80% rule, known as *hara hachi bu*, which means they stop eating when they feel 80% full, not stuffed. They gather around tables to eat slowly, with conversation and connection. They sip red wine in moderation. And perhaps, most importantly, they live with deep purpose and are anchored in close-knit communities where they feel loved.

It's a beautiful reminder that the way we live each day matters. You can create your own version of a Blue Zone, right where you are.

Harry, one of my greatest mentors, was still full of energy and a hint of mischief, well into his mid-seventies. He started a young family in his sixties and even dressed with a youthful flair. He never really "retired." Every morning, he would wake up at the crack of dawn with a project to build or a dream to chase. He was always eager to learn and try new things, and never afraid to change course if something wasn't working. He approached life with the curiosity of a teenager and an open heart for growth.

He once told me, "You need something to love, someone to play with, and something to look forward to." And he lived it. He had purpose.

Then there's my mother, now eighty-eight. She paints every day in her sunlit studio, still drives her little cornflower blue car she calls Egnor, and arrives at lunch wearing a pink floral dress with stories eager to spill from her lips. Her curiosity and strength have grown as she's aged. Her creativity keeps her sharp and vibrantly alive. But I've also seen the other side.

My father, after decades of purpose as a farmer, retired at eighty. And in the stillness that followed, the absence of animals to care for, land to walk, and sunrises to chase, his spark began to fade. Dementia followed quickly. I watched, heartbroken, as a once vibrant man became a shadow of himself. His story is a reminder that, without purpose, the body and spirit can begin to drift.

So, what will you choose for your next chapter? You get to choose. Your next chapter needs to be true to you. Maybe it looks like starting a walking group with friends. Maybe it's picking up that creative project you've always dreamed of. Maybe it's giving yourself full permission to rest, breathe, and savor.

Whatever you choose from here, whenever you can, do it with intention. Let it energize you. Let it reflect the woman you are now and the woman you're still becoming. Everything you've read in this book is now part of your toolkit. I mean that literally, too. Keep growing. Keep choosing you.

And, above all, stay connected. There's sisterhood here, too. We are in the middle of a quiet revolution, of women rising into their power and redefining what midlife can look like. We are in this together, and we are stronger together. So, share your story. Lean on each other. Celebrate the wins, no matter how small.

This is your moment. Write your next chapter with courage, honesty, and kindness. You've gained your wisdom, weathered the storms, and still have so much more to discover.

As you step into the unknown:

Let purpose lead.

Let wellness sustain you.

Let joy be your guide.

This is your moment to shine. To live the life you've always dreamed of. So, dream big. Dream boldly. Live a life you love, radiant and rooted in your power as the beautiful midlife woman you are.

Midlife isn't your ending. It's your awakening. This is your time. Step forward, radiant, unapologetic, and ready. Your second act is yours to claim.

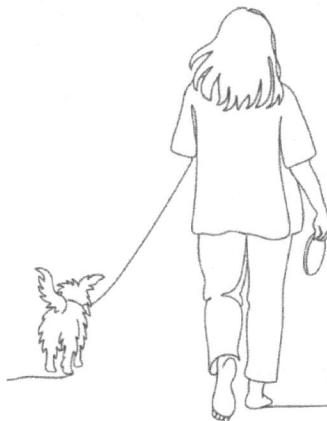

Appendix A

Additional Support and Reference

The chapters of this book are designed to guide you through midlife with warmth, clarity, and practical strategies you can begin using right away. But sometimes symptoms persist or questions come up that need more detail than what fits easily into the main flow of this book. That's what this appendix is for.

Here, you'll find deeper dives into conditions and supports that often overlap with menopause, such as thyroid disorders, chronic fatigue, autoimmune conditions, leaky gut, and SIBO. You'll also find reference-style notes on herbs, supplements, and other therapeutic tools that may be helpful.

Think of this section as a companion library. You don't need to read it cover to cover, but it's here to answer questions, give you practical options to discuss with your health care team, and reassure you that if your symptoms feel bigger than lifestyle tweaks, you're not imagining it.

The main book will walk you through the everyday practices that build strength and balance. This appendix is where you can turn when you want to explore specific conditions in more depth, track patterns, or take ideas into a conversation with your practitioner.

Gut Underlying Conditions

Leaky Gut

Also called increased intestinal permeability, leaky gut is one of those sneaky midlife saboteurs that often goes unnoticed. Your intestinal lining acts like a tightly woven mesh screen, designed to let nutrients through while keeping troublemakers out.

When estrogen levels drop, this barrier can weaken, allowing particles, such as toxins, microbes, and partially digested food, to slip through and trigger inflammation. This inflammation can show up not just in your belly, but across your whole body, as joint pain, brain fog, fatigue, or sudden food sensitivities that make you wonder why long-trusted foods now cause problems.

Signs to watch for: ongoing bloating, low energy, skin flare-ups, and digestive distress after eating previously well-tolerated foods.

Where to Start

Support your gut lining with nutrients, such as bone broth, collagen-rich foods, and zinc (pumpkin seeds are a simple source). L-glutamine, an amino acid found in cabbage, bone broth, and grass-fed beef can act like a mini repair kit for the intestinal wall. These foods nourish the gut lining, reduce inflammation, and improve absorption, all especially valuable at midlife when digestion may already be under extra stress.

SIBO: When Gut Bacteria Go Rogue

Small intestinal bacterial overgrowth (SIBO) occurs when bacteria that normally belong in the large intestine migrate into the small intestine. Hormonal changes that slow gut motility can make this more likely during menopause.

Typical signs: progressive bloating throughout the day (especially after carbs), abdominal cramping, and unpredictable bowel habits.

Where to Start

Managing SIBO usually requires professional support. Doctors may prescribe antibiotics, while some practitioners recommend herbal antimicrobials, such as berberine, oregano oil, neem, garlic extract, or allicin. At home, supportive habits can make a big difference: daily movement, mindful eating, and stress reduction all help keep gut motility flowing. Some health care professionals may also suggest spacing meals by three hours, reducing certain carbohydrates, or trialing a low-FODMAP diet.

These conditions can look and feel a lot like "just menopause." If your symptoms persist despite lifestyle changes, talk with your health care team. Getting the right tests and guidance can be the key to moving from surviving to thriving.

Underlying Conditions

Persistent fatigue, pain, or other symptoms in midlife are not always explained by hormonal shifts alone. Sometimes, they signal an underlying condition that requires medical attention. If your symptoms continue despite healthy lifestyle changes, it's important to seek support and consider further testing.

Below is an overview of common conditions that can overlap with, or be mistaken for, menopause symptoms:

Chronic Fatigue Syndrome (CFS)

Characterized by overwhelming exhaustion that does not improve with rest. Symptoms may include unrefreshing sleep, muscle and joint pain, poor concentration, and sensitivity to noise or light. Even simple daily tasks can feel monumental.

Hypothyroidism and Hashimoto's Thyroiditis

These thyroid disorders can slow digestion, mood, and energy. Signs may include weight gain despite healthy habits, feeling cold, bloating, low mood, or mental fog.

Requesting a full thyroid panel (TSH, Free T3, Free T4, and thyroid antibodies) can help with diagnosis.

Lupus and Other Autoimmune Conditions

Autoimmune disorders, such as lupus, rheumatoid arthritis, or Sjögren's syndrome, may present with joint pain, extreme fatigue, rashes, or sunlight sensitivity. Hormonal changes and stress can make symptoms more noticeable.

Polycystic Ovary Syndrome (PCOS)

A hormonal and metabolic condition that can cause irregular cycles, insulin resistance, weight gain, acne, and excess facial hair. PCOS symptoms often overlap with perimenopause and can affect long-term heart and metabolic health.

Fibromyalgia and Rheumatoid Arthritis

Fibromyalgia causes widespread muscle pain, poor sleep, and cognitive issues often described as "fibro fog." Rheumatoid arthritis leads to painful, swollen joints and morning stiffness. Both may flare and/or appear around midlife.

Multiple Sclerosis (MS)

A neurological condition in which the immune system damages the protective covering of nerves. Symptoms may include numbness, weakness, balance problems, or vision changes. Some women are diagnosed in midlife or notice symptom changes during perimenopause.

Energy-Smart Exercise Special Considerations

Midlife brings unique challenges such as burnout, thyroid changes, pelvic floor shifts, chronic pain, and autoimmune conditions. Movement can be one of your most powerful allies, but it needs to support your energy rather than drain it. Use this section as a guide to adapt your approach when your body needs extra care.

Burnout

When your nervous system is in overdrive, even a short walk can feel overwhelming.

What to avoid

- Loud gyms and overstimulating environments
- Compound or high-intensity training such as HIIT, bootcamps, or long cardio sessions
- Pushing through deep fatigue

- Relying heavily on caffeine to get through workouts

What to do instead

- Gentle isolated strength work, one muscle group at a time
- Restorative walks in nature without your phone
- Pilates or calming yoga with long exhalations
- Breathing, mobility, or stretching to soft music
- Guided relaxation or body scans

Hypermobility

Flexibility can become instability when connective tissue weakens.

What to avoid

- Deep passive stretching in already flexible joints
- Fast, momentum-driven movements
- Locking joints during strength training

What to do instead

- Controlled strength training using bands or light weights
- Slow Pilates with focus on core stability
- Active mobility instead of passive range of motion
- Balance and stability exercises

Chronic Pain

Pain is frustrating and unpredictable, but gentle movement helps keep your body resilient.

What to avoid

- High-impact activities such as running or jumping
- Forcing movement through pain
- Long or irregular sessions without pacing

What to do instead

- Short bursts of low-impact strength work
- Water-based movement, gentle cycling, or mini trampoline rebounding
- Gentle stretching, restorative yoga, or tai chi

Thyroid Imbalances

Hypothyroidism can leave you feeling sluggish. The right approach builds energy rather than drains it.

What to avoid

- Overtraining when energy is already low
- Long exhausting cardio
- Ignoring fatigue signals

What to do instead

- Gentle, consistent strength training
- Walks outdoors in natural light
- Planned recovery days and weeks

Insulin Resistance and Blood Sugar Swings

Hormone shifts can affect how your body handles sugar. Movement helps regulate blood sugar.

What to avoid

- Skipping meals or long fasting windows
- Excess cardio without fuel
- High-intensity training that overstresses the body

What to do instead

- Strength training two to three times per week
- Short walks after meals
- Daily gentle mobility or Pilates

Mood Disorders

Mood swings, low motivation, or overwhelm are common during perimenopause and menopause. Movement can shift your mental state.

What to avoid

- Punishing workouts that feel overwhelming
- Using exercise as a way to "fix" your body
- Exercising too hard and spiking cortisol
- Comparing yourself to your younger self or others

What to do instead

- Rhythmic movement such as walking, cycling, or dancing
- Strength training to rebuild confidence and focus
- Yoga, tai chi, or gentle stretching for emotional balance

Pelvic Floor Dysfunction

Weakened pelvic floor muscles can cause leaking, heaviness, or pain.

What to avoid

- Heavy lifting without pelvic floor activation
- Jumping, running, or high-impact exercise
- Ignoring early symptoms

What to do instead

- Daily stair walking
- Emptying your bladder before and during exercise
- Pilates for core and pelvic floor support
- Guided Kegel exercises with proper instruction

Autoimmune Conditions

Flare-ups can leave you drained, but the right movement reduces inflammation and supports recovery.

What to avoid

- High-intensity or high-impact training
- Ignoring signs of a crash
- Scheduling too much exercise without rest

What to do instead

- Short sessions of low-impact strength work
- Gentle cardio such as swimming or walking
- Breathwork, stretching, or yin yoga
- Complete rest on flare-up days

Final Note

Even if symptoms seem minor, persistent issues deserve proper evaluation. Many of these conditions are underdiagnosed in women, leading to unnecessary suffering. If something feels "off" in your body, trust your instincts, seek medical advice, and if needed, ask for referral to a specialist. Early support can make a significant difference.

Appendix B

Recommended Reading and Resources

Here are some of the books, experts, and tools that have inspired my journey and informed the guidance in *"Your Menopause Balance."* These aren't just references, you can use them as lifelines, inspiration to feel informed, empowered, and supported through midlife.

Brain Health and Hormones

- *The XX Brain* by Lisa Mosconi, PhD. A powerful, research-based look at how estrogen impacts memory, mood, and cognitive function, and how to protect and nourish your brain during menopause and beyond.

- *Outlive* by Peter Attia. Attia explores the science of not just prolonging life but also prolonging aliveness. Attia makes the crucial connection between overall health and relational health.

Hormones, Thyroid, and Healing

- *Medical Medium* by Anthony William, a book series including *Thyroid Healing*. Especially helpful when navigating chronic fatigue and hypothyroidism, with a focus on Epstein-Barr Virus and healing foods like kumara broth.

- "AUA/SUFU/AUGS 2025 Guidelines on Genitourinary Syndrome of Menopause" (GSM). Groundbreaking guidance for vaginal and urinary health in menopause, emphasizing how hormonal therapies, especially local ones, are safe and effective.

Movement and Menopause

- *The New Menopause* by Dr. Mary Claire Haver A refreshingly clear, evidence-based guide to navigating menopause with confidence. Dr. Haver breaks down hormone therapy, nutrition, and lifestyle strategies to help women make empowered, informed decisions about their midlife health.

- *Strength Training and Bone Health in Postmenopausal Women* by Thompson, J. A clinical look at why resistance training is so important in midlife to prevent osteoporosis and support longevity.

Nutrition and Gut Health

- *Wheat Belly* by Dr. William Davis. A groundbreaking look at how modern wheat contributes to inflammation, weight gain, gut issues, and hormonal disruption. Essential reading if you're exploring the link between gluten and midlife health.

- *The Role of Nutrition in Menopausal Health* by- Kim, S. A. comprehensive review of how to eat for hormonal balance, digestion, and energy during menopause.

Mindset, Motivation and Emotional Wellness

- *Loving What Is* by Byron Katie. Known as "The Work," it offers a powerful way to question stressful thoughts and shift inner dialogue. A transformative practice for reframing old beliefs, releasing self-judgment, and cultivating inner peace.

- *The Biology of Belief* by Dr. Bruce H. Lipton. A fascinating exploration of how our beliefs influence our biology. Lipton blends science and spirituality to show how mindset and perception can directly impact health, healing, and hormonal balance.

- *Awaken the Giant Within* by Tony Robbins. A practical and motivating guide to creating lasting change. His teachings on personal empowerment, daily rituals, and emotional mastery helped me move from burnout to balance during my own healing journey.

- *The New Menopause* by Dr. Mary Claire Haver. A bold and science-backed guide to navigating menopause with confidence. Dr. Haver offers clarity around hormone therapy, nutrition, and lifestyle—making the case for informed, empowered care

Lifestyle Inspiration

- *The Blue Zones* by Dan Buettner. An inspiring look into the world's longest-living communities and the lifestyle habits they share, natural movement, strong social ties, purposeful living, and fresh, unprocessed food. A powerful reminder that longevity is about daily rhythm, not rigid rules.

- *Unrest* (Netflix Documentary). Directed by Jennifer Brea. A deeply moving documentary that shines a light on chronic fatigue syndrome. Honest, emotional, and validating for anyone navigating invisible illness or seeking to be truly seen in their health journey.

Bibliography

Boardman, H.M.P., et al. (2015). Hormone therapy for preventing cardiovascular disease in postmenopausal women. Cochrane Database of Systematic Reviews. PMID: 25754617. Comprehensive analysis of HRT's role in heart disease prevention.

Conde, D.M., Verdade, R.C., Valadares, A.L.R., Mella, L.F.B., Pedro, A.O., & Costa Paiva, L. (2021). Menopause and cognitive impairment: A narrative review of current knowledge. World Journal of Psychiatry, 11(8), 412–428. PMID: 34513605 | DOI: 10.5498/wjp.v11.i8.412. Reviews the link between estrogen decline and cognitive changes in menopause.

Davis, S.R., et al. (2018). Understanding weight gain at menopause. Climacteric. PMID: 22978257. Breaks down how hormonal shifts influence fat redistribution and metabolism.

Erdélyi, A. (2023). The Importance of Nutrition in Menopause and Perimenopause — A Review. PMID: 38201856. Explores nutritional strategies to support hormone balance and metabolic health.

Gupta, S.K. (2022). Meditation, Mindfulness, and Mental Health: Opportunities, Issues, and Challenges. Hershey, PA: IGI Global. ISBN: 1799886824. Examines mindfulness as a tool for mental health support during midlife.

Hodis, H.N., et al. (2016). Vascular effects of early vs. late postmenopausal estradiol treatment. New England Journal of Medicine. PMID: 27028912. Showed early HRT initiation improves cardiovascular outcomes vs. delayed therapy.

Maeng, L.Y. (2023). Never fear, the gut bacteria are here: Estrogen and gut microbiome-brain axis interactions in fear extinction. PMID: 37207855. Highlights how estrogen influences gut-brain health and emotional resilience.

Maki, P.M. (2022). Brain fog in menopause: A health-care professional's guide for decision-making and counseling on cognition. PMID: 36178170. Provides clinical insights into managing menopause-related cognitive changes.

Massini, D.A., et al. (2022). The effect of resistance training on bone mineral density in older adults: A systematic review and meta-analysis. Healthcare, 10, 1129. DOI: 10.3390/healthcare10061129. Evaluates the impact of resistance training on bone density.

Ollie, V., et al. (2010). Risk of venous thrombosis with oral versus transdermal estrogen therapy among postmenopausal women. PMID: 20601871. Found that transdermal estrogen significantly lowers clot risk.

Peake, J.M., Tan, S.J., Markworth, J.F., et al. (2014). Metabolic and hormonal responses to isoenergetic high-intensity interval exercise and continuous moderate-intensity exercise.

American Journal of Physiology. PMID: 25096178. Explores exercise impacts on metabolism and hormone balance.

Pimentel, C. & Yu, D. (2024). Re-evaluating HRT Effects on Heart Disease Using Statistical Reanalysis. Source: arxiv.org (preprint). Confirms timing of HRT matters most using advanced modeling.

Schuman-Olivier, Z. (2020). Mindfulness and Behavior Change. PMID: PMC7647439. Explores how mindfulness supports long-term wellness habits.

---

www.ingramcontent.com/pod-product-compliance
Lightning Source LLC
Chambersburg PA
CBHW052120270326
41930CB00012B/2700